Nate's Bod in a Box program is different because it works! It works because I use it. I use it because it is simple. That is the entire story! Physically I see results MUCH more quickly than with free weights. And I am not experiencing injuries and setbacks like I was with free-weights and machines.

Leah B. -Madison, WI

Nate's blend of science, common sense, and humor makes his training program the best I've ever used.

Ross C. -Seattle, WA

Nate's Bod in a Box program stands out from the rest because it's all there for you – workouts and workout equipment. You can't take the squat rack with you outside, but you can take the bod in a box outside and change up the scenery of your workouts to keep it exciting. You can't make excuses with the Bod in a Box training.

Nicole B. -Glendale, AZ

Bod in a box is great because it has the simplicity of essential gear for workouts in a convenient pack. I feel mentally stronger when I work out and love the feeling after crushing it. Nate's training program is efficient, easy to follow, and you'll see improvement on a physical as well as mental level.

Maia F. -Phoenix AZ

Nate is an outstanding trainer, he is patient, well-educated and knowledgeable of the human body and the muscle system. Nate has made me aware of my strengths and provides continued support even outside of the workout.

Rick B. - Scottsdale, AZ

Best trainer ever! Nate makes training FUN. He taught me how train the right way to achieve the results that I wanted. I looked forward to every session with him. He is very professional and knowledgeable and committed to his clients and he knows how to get results. You will not be disappointed. Thank you, Nate!

Melissa K. - Phoenix, AZ

You will get results because Nate is a great motivator. His philosophy on health and fitness has forever changed the way I eat and live. I can honestly say that after using Nate's training I now get the best out of myself in the gym. He is why I lost 50 pounds in 4 months and because of the knowledge I got, I've been able to keep it off and lose more! THANKS NATE!

Matt E. - Tempe, AZ

Nate takes his profession seriously and expects results. He has a unique ability to provide intense workouts and have a sense of humor at the same time.

Larry T.

Nate is Amazing! He has completely turned my life around. I would never be where I am today if it weren't for him. Not only will you change your body, you change the way you feel about yourself! I am 100x more confident than I've ever been, he makes you realize the potential you have!

Lena G.

Nate is an amazing trainer! He is patient and intuitive to see what his clients need to be successful and adapts to meet their needs. I would highly recommend Nate to anyone looking to improve their fitness and get healthy! Thanks for always being there for me Nate!

Marmmett H. -Gilbert, AZ

Nate is the next generation of trainer in his ability to adapt to his clients at any level and any goal. His knowledge base keeps growing because he keeps trying to get better at his craft. He's a great trainer, and a great dude, and his sense of humor makes fitness fun again.

Carson K -Scottsdale, AZ

Technical, well read, and relatable, Nate Palmer makes functional fitness a nonstop, encouraging, goal-oriented journey that even appeals to those who hate the gym.

Kimberly Elliot -Ahwatukee, AZ

PASSPORT FITNESS

The No-Nonsense Guide To
Being In Shape No Matter
What City You Wake Up In

Nate Palmer III

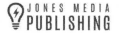
JONES MEDIA
PUBLISHING

Jones Media Publishing
10645 N. Tatum Blvd. Ste. 200-166
Phoenix, AZ 85028
www.JonesMediaPublishing.com

Printed in the United States of America

ISBN-13: 978-1-945849-48-0 paperback

CONTENTS

Section 1: Intro

I had walked for the better part of 20 minutes and still hadn't found the "perfect" place to set up my suspension strap. "You're just stalling," I thought to myself, as I spotted a serviceable tree about 30 yards away. There! That would work just fine.

As I walked toward the tree that would be my gym for the next 30 minutes, I noticed a small tienda (a little corner store with snacks and cheap beer) directly behind it with about nine men sitting around, drinking cerveza and talking.

No matter. It wasn't the first time I had an audience while doing oddly sexual bodyweight moves suspended from trees, beams, doors, or anything else I could find.

I set up my equipment, put some hard rock on the headphones, and started doing my workout, which was physically and metaphorically destroying me. I had literally just fallen on my face after a set of pushups that weren't normally difficult. Out of the corner of my eye, I noticed one of the men from the tienda walking over toward me, hiding one of his hands behind his back.

Shit. I was laying on the ground, tangled up in my strap, with no good escape route. My mind flashed back to all the decisions I'd made that brought me to this point.

My wife Lindsay and I had been traveling through Central and South America for about nine months. We had worked as tour guides on the Panama Canal, pig farmers in Ecuador, and school teachers in a suburb outside of Lima, Peru and had spent the remainder of the time exploring and adventuring

We had just arrived in a small town in the mountains of Peru called Huaraz after having taken an overnight bus from Lima, about an 8-hour journey. After getting lost on the way to our hostel several times, we dumped our stiff and tired bodies into our beds for a nap.

After waking up, I did what I always tried to do — a quick bodyweight workout to start my day off right.

The difference between where we were and the cities we had previously been in is that Huaraz had an elevation of about 9,500 feet, so between the massive elevation gain and the fact that we had spent the previous night on a smelly and cramped bus, the "easy" workout I was doing was crushing my soul.

I stared up at the approaching man as I tried to get my feet unhooked from the straps so that I could better fight him, or run away (probably run away though).

I was able to get to one knee as the approaching man got within a few feet of me. I don't want to brag about my karate skills, but let's just say that if he had wanted to stab me, there would have been very little I could have done to stop him.

Instead, from behind his back he produced a Cusquena – a cold Peruvian beer. In Spanish he said, "Hey amigo, don't exercise; drink a beer with us instead."

I did cut my workout short to drink a beer (or two) with my new friends, but simply getting out and doing some physical activity GREATLY prepared me for the rest of my time in Huaraz. The next day, we hiked a glacier at 15,000 feet, and the following day, we did a 9-hour trek that gained about 4,000 feet of elevation.

While many of my fellow hikers were dragging due to the high elevation, my lungs and muscles felt great because of the consistent workouts I had done over the previous months, as well as the brief high-

*elevation acclimation workout I had done despite
the protests from both body and mind.*

Beyond magazines promising fat loss and sweet
biceps in just minutes per day, exercise can have
profound effects on your physical and mental well-
being.

This isn't some well-kept secret by the upper echelon
of lizard people who run the country. This is real news,
and something that 10/10 people will tell you is true.

The main reason someone will stop getting results
or start to backslide is a lack of consistency. Short,
effective workouts make staying consistent easy. Not to
mention, they allow your body to utilize the additional
calories from that delicious pasta you had at dinner.

Carrying more muscle around than the average
person will also ensure that you recover more quickly
from those inevitable off-plan days that happen in our
busy lives.

Yes, life happens. But consistent daily exercise is one
of the things that will help keep your body and mind
sharp regardless of the struggles or successes of the
day. Quick, effective workouts will also help you feel
your best and get the most out of your travel without
needing a vacation every time you return home.

STOP FALLING OFF YOUR ROUTINE

The best predictor of long-term success in your health and fitness is consistency. The main reason that this book will not be considered for Gwyneth Paltrow's YouTube book review is because we refused to lie and tell you that the secret to health and fitness is yak butter and taking small breaths.

The more consistent we are, and the more we can make exercise just another thing on our schedule for the day, the better our results will be. When everyone else is making New Year's resolutions (again) or Googling, "how to get a bikini body lol" (again) you'll be fine, because you have been consistent for the last several presidential administrations.

If vacation went from something that derailed our progress to being a non-event in regard to our general fitness, we'd be on our way to a body that is lean for life.

.... BUT YOU ALREADY KNOW ALL THIS.

That's the thing. We all know we *should* be exercising and eating healthy. Beyond that, we feel good when we're working out!

But it's hard to know exactly *what* we need to be doing. Additionally, what happens when we're at a strange hotel in Paris, Texas, there's no gym, the pool

5

is closed, and its 99 percent humidity outside with 100 percent mosquitos?

Plus, we're tired from a long flight, we've only eaten airplane peanuts and coffee for the past 8 hours, and we've got a meeting to prepare for.

When life takes a big, steamy dump on your plans, what do you do?

In this book, I'll share some things that have worked for me during a full year of traveling: And by traveling, I mean 255 hours on buses, 55 hostels, 42 cities, 23 flights, and 7 hospitals. I'll also throw in some strategies I've gleaned from friends and clients who take 30-plus work trips each year.

This book is not meant to be a direct blueprint for you to follow, but rather a collection of helpful information and tips that you can take from as you need, to create a routine that fits your lifestyle.

If you're on the road half the time, you'll need different strategies than the person that travels two times per year for a month at a time.

Bruce Lee once said, "Take what is useful. Discard what is not." He borrowed from a lot of different martial arts disciplines and created a new system that he believed to be superior to others. Called Jeet Kune Do, it was a combination of battle-tested techniques and some of his own.

My goal with this book is to help you create your own Jeet Kune Do.

Whether you travel internationally for work several times per month, or are just going to visit your Aunt Margret for the holidays, you need to build the system that works for your lifestyle to stay fit, healthy, and strong.

Your health doesn't stop existing just because you're out of the house, so let's grow up and stop pretending that a 6-year-old's birthday party is a good excuse to throw your goals in the metaphorical trash compactor.

Onward!

Section 2: Why you should care

Daily training, especially while traveling, sharpens your body and mind while allowing you to be more present for the important aspects of your life and job.

Ok, so yeah, *duh*. Working out daily is important.

But why the hell does that matter to you, and how can we convert that knowledge into new consistent habits and behavior?

In June of 2017, I brought a group of people down to Lake Gatun in Panama to visit a place that I had worked at for 6 months as a jungle guide. The focus of the trip was not only adventure and exploration, but activity, exercise, and fitness. And rum. We explored plenty of rum.

We woke up early each morning and did something active to start the day off right. The best days always start with morning yoga, a light-suspension trainer workout, or paddle boarding through the jungle islands that surround the Panama Canal.

Then we grabbed breakfast and headed toward whatever adventure I had planned for the day. One day, we did a day-long jungle trek upriver, bushwhacking our way with a machete when the trail was blocked by fallen trees.

The second day, we paddled kayaks six miles from the interior of the country out to the Caribbean Sea, to an old fort that had been occupied by Captain Henry Morgan, the Welsh Pirate who invaded Panama City, raped, murdered, and pillaged so hard, that they literally had to rebuild the city in a new location. I mean, I've left hotel rooms in bad shape, but I've never partied so hard that it was necessary to rebuild an entire metropolitan area. Anyways.... we grabbed bikes at the fort and rode another 12 miles back to base camp.

Each day was dedicated to activity and adventure – incredibly rewarding and fun, but extremely rare in normal life.

Let's face it, unless you're coming on one of my retreats, you're probably not going to get this insane amount of activity on a regular vacation, much less that work trip to Houston you do four times per year.

I'm not trying to shame you though. Far from it.

Every trip we take has a purpose. Whether it's kicking back with the family or trying to get new business, we don't travel *just because.*

The exercise you do should build toward that goal, not detract from it.

So how does daily exercise support your lifestyle?

5 Reasons for Daily Workouts

Daily workouts are the best way to look and feel your best for your entire life. Everyday exercise has incredible benefits beyond just having great arms. Not only will you look better, you'll also have:

- More endorphins
- Higher mental energy
- More physical energy
- Food goes to muscles instead of fat
- Metabolic snowballing
- Decreased chance of "falling off the wagon"

Endorphins

Endorphins is a word that is thrown around, but little understood. Science tells us that endorphins are "endogenous opioid neuropeptides that are produced by the central nervous system and the pituitary gland."

But that doesn't mean much, unless you happen to be a neuro-scientist or a total nerd.

All you need to know about these delicious molecules floating around in your brain juice is in the name. "Endo" comes from *endogenous*, which means "inside", and "orphin" comes from *morphine*, which is a drug used for pain relief. So basically, these are naturally produced opioids that your brain makes to help you feel great and turn off your pain receptors.

Endorphins are naturally produced by kissing, exercising, and laughing. That's why you should strive to do these things daily.

MENTAL ENERGY

Along with endorphins, working out can often bring a clarity or mental focus to your day.

Especially when starting the day with even a quick workout or movement session, you can focus your attention on the task at hand while your subconscious goes to work on solving the problems of the day for you.

Most of my best ideas and solutions come when I'm no longer focused on the activity, but doing something else, like taking a shower or working out.

Especially if there's a specific issue that's been on your mind recently, it's important to give your conscious mind a break and let your subconscious work through the details.

Beyond solving problems, exercise will increase blood flow to the brain and give you physical and mental energy for the day ahead. Recent studies have shown that individuals with a higher level of fitness had an ability to allocate more focus to external tasks, which made them able to do more "thoughtful" work in less time, and more efficiently.

Exercise was also linked to "neuroplasticity", which is a fancy word for being able to respond better and faster to the stimuli of the day.

The faster you can respond, the better prepared you'll be for animal attacks and avoiding life threatening injuries.

One of the places I worked in Panama was a small organic farm on a remote island in the archipelago of Bocas Del Toro. My responsibilities included: administering vaccines to angry bulls, cutting down and carrying a massive cedar tree from deep in the jungle out to a tiny boat to bring back home for construction, and burning the trash.

While there were always adventures on the island, the most harrowing one (and the one that sent me to the hospital) was lighting a trash fire on a large pile of brush that had been soaked overnight by a jungle thunderstorm. The owners of the farm had left for the day on the single boat, leaving my wife and I to work on building the new treehouse addition.

13

Since the big pile of trash was wet, I decided to liberally use some gasoline to "coax" the trash fire into existence. What I didn't realize was that the gas on the island was all unrefined. This means that there's no oil in it, which makes it more stable, and keeps it from evaporating. A 5-gallon bucket of unrefined gasoline will evaporate in under two hours if left uncovered.

What this meant for me was that when I leaned in with a lighter to start the fire, instead of a slow build, the entire pile of garbage, wood, and cardboard erupted in my face, causing 2nd degree burns from my neck all the way down my legs.

My wife was watching from a few feet away and said that the flames engulfed my body and threw me backwards. All I remember is hitting the ground and thinking back to elementary school "stop, drop, and roll" drills. And roll I did, not realizing for a minute that I was literally burned from head to toe. That's one reason that I have 7 hospital visits on my travel resume. With a bit of extra neuroplasticity, I probably would have been fine!

This makes you sharper when you have to tap into your high school spanish skills, bring your A-game to an important presentation, or concentrate on lighting an enormous fire without causing several hospital visits.

PHYSICAL ENERGY FOR ACTIVITIES

Despite how you felt after your first or second workout, exercise will build your overall energy stores for the future. This "battery" of overall energy will increase in size, allowing you to have more physical and mental energy for clients, family, and mental processing.

This is backward from how most people view training – as an expense. But it's actually an investment in your future abilities and energy.

The more you invest in daily workouts and slowly begin to build your battery, the more energy you'll have to invest, in exercise, meetings, activities, and life.

President Trump has a theory that I think many Americans share when it comes to physical activity. He subscribes to the "all you've got is all you'll have" mentality, in which you basically have 1000 points to spend during your life. In this model, exercising, drinking, or summiting Everest would decrease your lifetime energy stores by several points. Not to mention that spring break in Cabo, where I would have lost 29 points in two days. This philosophy would mean that doing formal exercise is the worst time and energy investment ever.

But that's simply not true. Energy levels can vary wildly through your life depending on level of physical

15

fitness, overall health, and behaviors. Ask any 20-year-old who weighs 400-plus pounds how much energy they have daily, and you'll find that most morbidly obese people don't feel like taking a quick walk. Ever.

As you adjust to an increased energy expenditure daily, your body will accommodate you by helping you wake up with more energy, have more sustained vigor during the day, and you'll also get the benefit of sleeping harder.

Our bodies are incredibly smart and can adapt to anything we throw at them. But they don't like to change unless we give them a good reason. Most often that reason is survival related.

This is why exercise works for getting stronger. If you don't want to get crushed by a heavy bench press, your body must prioritize growing new muscle and training it to be strong. It's a simple survival mechanism, but can be powerful when harnessed effectively.

We live in a first-class society, where being biggest and strongest is no longer the primary driver of success and procreation. While many people argue that this means that we need less fitness in our lives, I believe that to live an above-average life we need to train our bodies to be physically capable, strong, and energetic.

This also prepares us for the coming zombie apocalypse, where those who shirked their training will get eaten first.

FOOD GOES TO MUSCLES

One of the greatest things about working out is building muscle. Muscle makes you harder to kill, keeps your joints strong and injury free, and make you look great in a tank top.

When you exercise, you break down your muscles, which then require fuel to rebuild. The food you eat breaks down into the necessary pieces (providing you're eating food that's good for you) and helps to construct new muscle tissue.

The more you exercise and the more muscle you have, the higher your daily metabolic burn will be. When we travel, we don't always get to eat the healthiest foods. That's a fact of life. Having a higher metabolism gives us a "nutritional airbag" to negate the issues that many people feel after stuffing their face full of burgers and fries.

If you're exercising, when you accidentally grab a third serving of pie at the all-inclusive buffet, you can rest assured that many of those calories will be allocated for energy within your muscles rather than sent to long-term fat storage.

17

NATE'S HOT TIP

Nutritional Airbag – a *phrase I just made up to describe having a higher metabolism based on lifestyle and activity. You'll know you have nutritional airbags installed when your weight basically stays the same even after a vacation, or you can return to your pre-Thanksgiving weight after 5-7 days.*

The more exercise we can do during our lives, the higher our metabolism will be and the more muscle we'll have.

"But Nate!" you say. "I don't want to have too much muscle!"

Well, Jessica, you've probably driven your car for more hours than you've ever put in on the treadmill, and you're in no danger of becoming a NASCAR driver.

METABOLIC SNOWBALLING

When you work out hard, you get an "afterburn" effect that helps you continue to burn calories for the following 24-48 hours. The more intense the workout, the higher the afterburn effect.

When you start stringing together workouts multiple times per week, the afterburn effect seems to snowball. This gentle increase to your metabolism doesn't add up to a ton of extra calories burned, but over time, it's a difference of thousands of calories per year.

Most of the time it's difficult for us to squeeze in intense daily workouts. Either we overdo it slightly and get sore, or we just can't motivate ourselves to push it day after day.

But even just a 30-minute walk can add to this metabolic snowball effect. Especially when just starting off, or in a high-stress time in life, alternating between intense workouts and low-intensity cardio can be the better option.

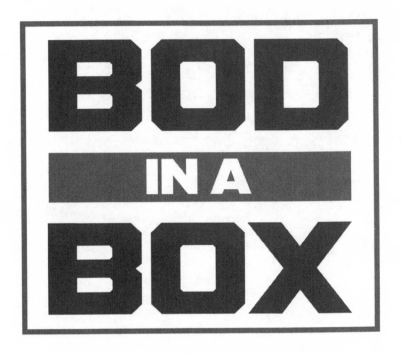

To get a FREE copy of the workout program that I've used successfully with hundreds of clients, visit:

http://bodinabox.com/free

Learn:

- The home workout you can do anywhere
- The best exercises you can do in a hotel room
- The right pace for a 15-minute workout that will give you results
- The one exercise you need to be doing every day

Section 3: Calling You Out

"The hotel gym is crappy."

"Ugh, late client meetings."

"Too many glasses of wine the night before."

Any of this sound familiar? These are called "excuses," and Webster defines them as, *"a reason put forward to justify a fault or an offense."*

Your Excuses Are Trash.

Human beings are unique in our ability to walk for hours at a time, post to Snapchat, and justify any type of bad behavior.

Life is going to happen to us no matter what. There will always be something on the periphery trying to detract from our goals, take our time, or otherwise occupy us. There are several things (read: Facebook) tugging at my attention right now, trying to get me to stop writing. The point is, there are **always distractions** and **always excuses**.

They never go away, they never get easier, and there's never a perfect time. *Wah, wah, wah.*

The way I see it, we have two options. We can accept the fact that we are tiny pinballs batted about by metaphysical elements outside of our control in the universe, or we can rebel against this powerless philosophy and take control.

If you're still subscribing to the first philosophy, the rest of this book is gonna be a tough read. You should probably give it away to someone else, and tell them that it was written like shit, and that the author had a bad attitude.

Taking control sounds great, right? But here's what that means.

CHANGE YOUR MINDSET – CHANGE YOUR BODY

Everything is your fault.

Yup, you own it.

You own everything.

Late again for work? Nope, it wasn't that there was a car accident, it was because you didn't leave early enough or take a better route.

Coworker didn't finish the work they were supposed to do? You must not have communicated clearly enough and followed up.

Yes, there will always be late nights and early meetings. There will always be a company credit card and a client dinner. And you'll always have 31 flavors to choose from at Baskin-Robbins.

A lot of things are outside of our control, but I have yet to meet a person who doesn't waste at least 30 minutes every day on TV, social media, or _____ (fill in your bad habit of choice here).

No matter the hand we're dealt, we always have options. And once you realize that you're in control, you can make decisions based on that information.

Excuse: I only have 15 minutes before I need to meet clients.

- Option One: Do 15 minutes of movement and stretching to prepare your body and mind to sit in another meeting.
- Option Two: Lay on the bed with a pillow over your face, dreading the thought of pretending to be nice for three consecutive hours.

Excuse: I'm 7 hours behind because of jet lag.

- Option One: Automatically assume the time zone and supplement with caffeine and alcohol to "prepare" your body for its new lifestyle.
- Option Two: Whine to co-workers all day about how tired you are.

23

Excuse: Clients taking longer than I planned to learn the new software.

- Option One: Assume you're not doing all you can do to teach them effectively, and upgrade your game to better serve them.
- Option Two: Assume all the clients are all scramble-brains and will never learn anything.

Excuse: Holiday season got me all hot and bothered over baked goods and spiked eggnog.

- Option One: Ensure that you're making time for your workouts every day, eat lots of fruits and veggies early in the day, and be moderate at dinner.
- Option Two: Complain to whoever will listen about how these cookies are going straight to your ass.

This type of decision-making is difficult, and requires action and self-reflection, but will serve you well for the rest of your life.

While this is not a self-help book because I'm incredibly unqualified to help you with anything other than getting ripped, healthy, and happy – this **"growth mindset"** is prevalent in anyone who's ever transformed or changed their body.

Think about that...

Consistency > Everything

The Truth About Accountability

For a 3-year period, I worked for a massive health club that was also running one of the longest and most elaborate weight-loss studies in the world. The study has been running for more than 30 years, and boasts an impressive 50 percent weight-loss maintenance record.

The global average hovers right around 5 percent. That means 95 percent of the people who lose weight will regain it within 2 years.

What's so special about this program that they have rates 10 times higher than the running average?

The Program is an expensive and all-encompassing, medically supervised program that requires:

- *3 sessions with a personal trainer per week*
- *1 session with a dietician per week*
- *1 session with a counselor per week*
- *1 session with a support group per week*
- *1 doctor appointment per month*
- *A 12-stage elimination diet that gets rid of all inflammatory and allergenic foods before slowly reintroducing foods to the system*

You're probably thinking, "Uh yeah, I could definitely lose weight on that program."

And you're right. You definitely would!

But the catch isn't the weight loss, it's the maintenance. Remember, a lot of people lose weight before putting it right back on.

What separates the 50 percent who keep it off from the 50 percent who don't? Didn't they all go through the same program?

(If you think that "eat more veggies" is a pretty good health secret, then this one is really gonna blow you away.)

Consistency.

The people that continued to maintain the consistency they had built into their daily habits were the ones who maintained their results.

For some people, that meant playing racquetball a few days per week on top of their workouts. For some, it was finding an exercise class they liked. Others established an easy-to-follow home workout routine with a few key pieces of equipment.

NATE'S HOT TIP

"Exercise" in this context doesn't mean a light walk with your besties in matching velour joggers. I'm talking about a sweat sesh, where the heart rate goes up and you might be having a hard time getting enough air. The kind where when you're done, you are DONE.

The type of exercise that they used was LESS important than the fact that they were doing exercise.

A Health Mindset is a Lifetime Goal – It doesn't turn off because you're at a hotel

People who went through The Program mentioned above would also have another epiphany about their health as a "forever thing."

I'll never forget the day a new client came in and started crying during our initial session.

He was an ex-collegiate athlete with National Championships to his name, but when I asked him why he was in the program, he broke down.

"I just never thought about the fact that there are no do-overs," he said.

He went on to tell me that after a successful athletic career he decided to, "take a year off" from health and fitness. What started as a mental break quickly became 2 years, then 5, then 22.

At the end, he was able to look back and see how much his career, his marriage, and his body had suffered from the "time-off" mentality.

The truth is, there is no time off.

27

You get one body and you're stuck with it forever. This is good news to some and bad news to others.

The good news is that you're going to have your same body one year from now. How it looks, and feels is up to you and your actions.

The bad news is exactly what my client said. There are NO do-overs.

THE 80/20 PRINCIPLE

Just because there are no do-overs doesn't mean there are no beers, wings, or cheesecake.

A world without hot wings is a world I'm not interested in, thank you very much.

That's why the 80/20 principle works well for me in keeping a healthy mindset front and center, while still allowing for let's say ... Cinnabon. Or 6 beers.

If 80-90 percent of my diet is real food that I cook myself, the 3 meals I eat out with clients won't make or break my progress.

If you nail your workouts 80 percent of the time, and 20 percent of the time just show up and punch the clock, or simply skip the workout in favor of a walk later, you'll still get better long-term results than most people who step foot in a gym.

The Magic Pill

Everyone wants a magic pill to help them lose weight fast, get ripped abs, and grow a giant dong.

But regardless of whether the results come fast or slow, time always seems to pass.

Many people make the mistake of trying to have health and fitness occupy 100 percent of their attention for 3 weeks and end up burning out.

But if your health is always a constant low-grade point of attention for you, how much easier is it to make good choices, rather than switching to a full vegan diet and doing bikram CrossFit?

The reality for anyone is that any *good* goal is at least a year-long project.

No matter how long it takes you to reach that goal, maintaining it for a full year helps your body to "lock in" changes through a shift in metabolism and a weight set point.

But most of us miss the point and aim for a better beach body in 3 weeks, knowing full well we're going to drink gallons of daiquiris at the resort and order room service at 3 a.m.

Yes, vacations are fun, and staying up too late is an important part of life, but that lifestyle isn't conducive to a healthy mind and body.

29

Keys to the Kingdom

Everyone's "why" is different.

When I was spending most of my time training individuals, it was always interesting to hear what people's goals were.

I started my career not in fitness, but in sales, and was trained to always dig into people's reasons for making a purchase to find out what their true goals were. Like an onion, it's important to peel back the metaphorical layers to find the truth.

One Friday afternoon, I had a new client assessment with a woman who came in requesting some information on training for a 5K race.

I was feeling a little lazy, and almost opted for just talking her through the steps of being ready for a short race like that. It's not super hard, and the training wouldn't be difficult. Instead, I kept asking her for more info – why she wanted to run a 5K, had she been a runner before, how she would look and feel in six months if all our training went 100 percent to plan.

Suddenly, she broke down and confessed to me that a 5k wasn't that important, but rather she wanted to have the physique of one of her friends who also happened to be a runner (as well as a cyclist and suspension-training enthusiast).

I dug deeper, and she told me that her new interest in fitness had come as a result of her overhearing a conversation between her husband and his friend where he had casually let it slip that he wasn't physically attracted to her like he used to be.

Wow.

Yes, that's hurtful and deeply emotional, but the contrast is powerful.

To go from a goal of running a 5K to the *real* goal of rekindling the romance in her relationship, which do you think is going to provide a deeper commitment after the initial allure of training wears off?

The point is that we all have different goals. Our lives, relationships, and career are going to take precedence over the goal of doing 100 pushups in a row.

BUT, no matter what your life goals are, daily movement is an important piece.

From nailing a board meeting with the company executives, hiking at 10,000 feet without feeling spent, or imbibing more than you should without seeing the consequences on the scale the next day, exercise is an integral piece in the lives of thousands of extremely successful men and women across the globe and throughout the ages. Make it a non-negotiable habit, and experience the success that comes in the rest of your life.

Section 4. Travel Considerations

While daily exercise is still king, there are a million other little decisions that you're faced with on a daily basis that affect how you look, feel, and perform on the road.

These "little" decisions add up to big portions of your lifestyle, which can have a immense impact on your energy levels and the way your body looks and feels.

Most of the traveling that my wife and I did through Central and South America was on a bus, but there were certain places that just wasn't a good option.

The Darien Gap is a big section of jungle between Panama and Colombia. It's the piece that separates Central and South America, and even though there's land there, it's considered one of the most dangerous areas in the world.

Filled with pirates, drug cartels, and human traffickers, the Darien Gap is a lawless and perilous zone that even the police and military avoid. So even though we had set out in search of adventure, we decided to take the safe bet and fly from Panama into Medellin, Colombia.

The Panama airport is like most airports – devoid of healthy food options. Even more here, because everything that had even a semblance of health was deep-fried or coated in sugar.

But after a flight delay and a travel mix-up that involved me talking the attendant into letting me behind the airline computer to forge bus tickets in MS Paint to avoid violating the terms of our visa, we were hungry!

Since not eating isn't an option most of the time, we had to adapt. We ended up buying a whole roasted chicken and a whole papaya which we cut up and ate – seeds and all! (Papaya seeds are a superfood that can help with gut health).

We finished our meal by each downing a bottle of water, because you never know what you're going to get on the actual airplane.

Not to say this is the best option all the time, or that we couldn't have been more prepared, but we were able to find a serviceable option that helped us stay healthy and full during a stressful time when it would have been easy to just eat fried plantains. Mmmmmm good.

A big part of traveling for work is the actual *travel* part.

It's great to take pictures in front of a waterfall in Costa Rica, but no one takes any pictures of the unglamorous part of the adventure where your portly neighbor falls asleep on your shoulder in the cramped van on the 3 hour drive out to the waterfall. Nobody posts about the stiff lower backs and the jet lag on Instagram, yet it's a very real part of the lifestyle.

This goes double for those of us who travel for work on a weekly basis. We have plenty of experience with travel time, TSA pat-downs, and Uber drivers that *just can't* seem to find your hotel.

Because health is a full-time mindset, how do we stay in the zone during full-travel days?

In this section we'll talk about some strategies you can use to inject a little bit of health and fitness into your life on the go.

I'll show you some strategies that many of my clients have used successfully – without having to do yoga in the security line.

How to Get Off the Plane Feeling Good

If you want to get off the plane feeling good, you need to structure your pre-flight and post-flight rituals in a way that makes sense for you.

Things that are important to consider are hydration, stretching, how you sit or sleep on the plane, staying healthy during a trip in germ-filled metal tube, and making sure you have the right equipment to have a pleasant flight based on how long it's going to be.

These are a few of the millions of little choices that come our way every day, and while bringing a neck pillow with you won't give you abs, it will be easier to get the daily exercise you need when you don't feel stiff and sore for 48 hours following a flight.

Hydration

Planes and hotels are stuffy. The air is dry, recycled, and you're breathing in air that the sick person over in 14B just finished exhaling.

The air on planes will dry out your sinuses, and cause you to be dehydrated even if you're drinking your normal amount of water because of the elevation and poor air quality.

A decrease in hydration will also produce a marked decrease in energy and strength. A 3 percent drop in your hydration can cause up to a 30 percent drop in

36

strength. This is the difference between benching 200lbs and 140lbs!

It's that important!

Not only that, but when we burn fat, most of the time it leaves our body through exhalation, and in order to be most effective at that, we need to make sure we're breathing out moist air. The only way to do this is to stay properly hydrated always.

If you're taking a flight longer than 90 minutes, sorry, but that little 6-ounce glass of water isn't going to cut it. You're going to need a water bottle.

In fact, one of the habits that the leanest

NATE'S HOT TIP

Hydrating beverages:

- *Water*
- *Coconut Water*
- *Gatorade (be careful of high sugar content though)*
- *Tea*
- *Bonus: Electrolyte powder. This is a great option if you're sweating a lot or just don't like drinking a lot of straight water. Find a low- or zero-calorie electrolyte powder to add to drinks. Lemon-lime or citrus flavors are always best. Always.*

Dehydrating Beverages:

- *Coffee*
- *Soda (honestly just stop drinking soda, it has no redeeming qualities)*
- *Alcohol*
- *Bonus: If you're drinking alcohol on the plane or at a bar, make sure to go 1 for 1 with a glass of water. That will help keep the hangover at bay, keep you hydrated, and help the alcohol absorb faster.*

37

people in the world have is keeping a water bottle with them at all times.

Pack an empty one with you through security, or fill it up when you leave the house and try to finish it before you get to the body scanner. Live on the edge!

In addition to bringing a water bottle on the plane, it's a good strategy to pound 24 ounces of water before and after your flight to negate dehydration. You'll feel better, I promise. Just try it.

This is the same advice I give people to recover from 8 hours of sleep at night with no water – fill up a bottle with 24-32 ounces and pound it when you get up. That's a great way to reset, and to make sure that you're hydrated going into your day.

Don't like to chug water? Ummm, I guess just sip it then? Sounds boring.

POSTURE

When sitting in an airplane, the easiest way to have great posture is by sitting up straight in the position you'd like to stay in, then cinching your seatbelt around your waist tightly to hold you in this position. Add in a neck pillow, and you're ready for a healthy hibernation.

What to Order

If you're trying to get off the plane feeling good, you're going to want to have at least three or four Jack and Cokes while you're on the plane. But if you're trying to get off the plane feeling great, I would advise sticking with water, or ordering tomato juice, just because of the vitamins and minerals. Plus, it's not a thing I drink daily, which makes it a nice treat.

Ordering food on an airplane – or even in the airport – can be tricky because there are not a lot of good options. If you didn't prepare and bring snacks and healthy food options with you, just opt for the highest-protein option that they offer in flight.

Protein is more satiating, so it will keep you full longer. It also aids in muscle recovery and is very difficult for your body to convert into fat.

Don't order soda. We all know that sodas aren't good for us. Choosing to slurp down some dirty corn-syrup water is one of the silliest things we can do when traveling because it's dehydrating and loads your body with sugar.

Sugar increases your insulin, which makes your body crave more sugar – a vicious cycle.

This is a horrible idea if you want to set yourself up for success moving forward. You don't want to start a work trip feeling bloated with no energy.

The ONLY exception is if nausea is a problem for you, then order a ginger ale. This is the only soda you should ever get. Sometimes, the small amount of ginger will cut the edge of the nausea.

I get it though, we've all been on that flight to vegas with three of our friends, where we end up trying to talk the flight attendant into giving us six or seven bottles of tiny liquor apiece rather than our allotted one or two. And those times are important as well, but if you travel extensively for work, or if you're trying to travel and feel your best, I would highly recommend against in-flight drinking.

Drinking sets you up for failure in that it lowers your inhibitions, and you'll be even more likely to go into the terminal and grab the nachos rather than eating something healthy.

ABSOLUTE NECESSITIES FOR COMFORTABLE TRAVEL:

- A neck pillow to make sure that you're not getting off with a stiff neck, especially if you're going to fall asleep.
- Noise-canceling headphones that you can listen to some music and not hear that baby down the aisle cry the entire flight.
- An eye mask, or beanie that can be converted into an eye mask.

- Water bottle – collapsible is a good call for the flight so you can fill it after you clear security, but anything with a lid will work.
- Healthy snack
- Kindle or eReader
- Emergen-C
- Phone-battery charger pack
- Sweatshirt/scarf

How to Tweak Your Training if You Strength Train

Flying can be a non-issue for some, but often, being locked in a cramped, seated position for hours at a time can leave frequent travelers with a stiff lower back, neck, or just general feelings of tightness.

For that reason, there are a few types of exercises that I tend to avoid a day or two before and after a flight.

If we train hard before a long travel day, there's a much higher chance that you'll feel super stiff leaving the plane, and that will reduce the chance that you'll want to do any exercise when you arrive.

After they return from a trip, I always have my clients avoid heavy spinal-loading exercises for at least 24 hours. This means heavy back squats, deadlifts, overhead presses, or cleans.

Those exercises will always be there, and I find that it's more beneficial to train the core directly or do a full bodyweight training program the day leading up to and returning from a trip.

Avoiding all exercise is silly because with the right movements performed correctly, we can strengthen the lower back and core to ensure that we leave the plane feeling great.

Avoid:

Heavy Leg Day.

If you generally do full-body workouts or at least train legs frequently enough that you don't get sore anymore, go ahead. But if you're the type that does legs once per week, and typically do some heavy squatting, deadlifting, or other compound movements, restructure your week so that you have *at least* two days of rest before sitting in a travel prison, errr plane seat, for hours at a time.

If you must do legs, stick to single-leg exercises that spare the lower back. Lunges, single-leg deadlifts, step-ups, and Bulgarian split-squats are great alternatives that will leave your legs sore, but your lower back feeling good.

Olympic Lifts.

When you use a ton of explosive force to move a barbell, the whole body has to be working in harmony to accelerate and decelerate the weights correctly. Most people are not training to be actual Olympic lifters, so there's no point to forcing your body to move heavy weights explosively if your body is still recovering from a lot of sitting or traveling.

Live to lift another day.

If you're hell-bent on Olympic lifting or doing your CrossFit WOD, you can easily sub kettlebell swings or high pulls for the more traditional Olympic lifts.

Do Train:

Just because you shouldn't do heavy squats or cleans within 2 days of big trips doesn't mean that you shouldn't train at all.

In fact, training the day before or the day of a long flight can help you feel better, stronger and healthier when you get off the plane. Make sure you're setting yourself up for success by working specific muscles and movement patterns.

Core.

Specifically training the *ANTI* movements. This means anti-flexion (planks) anti-extension (hollow-body holds), and anti-rotation (side planks and single-arm carries).

These types of exercises are challenging, but also lead to a better awareness of the body, and can also keep the back 30-50 percent more stable for up to 12 hours.

Upper Body.

Training the upper body is always a great option before a trip because you look more intimidating to fellow passengers, which will result in getting the use of both armrests as well as the endorphins from exercise without additional lower-back tightness.

Be careful of overdoing a chest workout though. Hammering the bench press, then sitting with poor posture for a few hours is a great way to wake up super sore!

Cardio.

Cardio is always a non-offensive choice that can be done directly before or after a trip without worrying about overdoing it.

It's a great way to get some blood flowing, burn a few calories, and put your head in the right place before leaving, as well as a good way to get your body back into the groove after getting back.

One of the best ways to avoid the feeling of jet lag is to immediately do some light cardio upon arriving at your destination. This can be as simple as going for a walk or a jog, and as a bonus you get to see more of the area that you're staying in.

How to Recover from a Big Trip

There are certain recovery protocols I use with myself and clients who have returned from a trip feeling slightly under the weather.

You know the feeling: Slightly plugged up through the sinuses, feeling a little like Quasimodo, and maybe that knee is acting up again.

No worries, just take it easy and follow these rules.

No Heavy Spinal Loading

If you get back from a 24-hour turnaround and jump right back into the gym to max out your squats, you might be fine, but you're also asking for an injury.

Because of the change in pressure, lack of sleep, and the fact that you've been sitting cramped up in an airplane seat for hours, your spine just isn't ready to handle the same load you would have been fine to do otherwise.

Instead, opt for a session that doesn't involve max weight or reps, then come back to your heavy lifting the next day. A yoga session is a great option, but at least make sure you spend double the amount of time on your warmup the first day back to your workout routine.

45

HEALTH INSURANCE

When I get back home I like to go through my nutritional insurance policy, which involves taking a few key supplements that enhance the immune system, improve sleep, and leave me feeling good for the following day.

1. Start with a big glass of water. Somewhere between 24-32 ounces will do the trick.
2. Then take 3000—5000 ius of Vitamin D (international units. A vitamin D pill is generally 2000-5000 ius.)
3. Mix a green-superfood supplement (usually a powder packed with your daily recommended dose of veggies) with a packet of Emergen-C, in water, and chug, chug, chug.
4. Finally, put 1-2 tablespoons of apple cider vinegar, in a glass of water with the juice from a lemon. Drink this before bed and upon rising.

Repeat this protocol for 1-3 days depending on how you're feeling. This is also my "avoid getting a cold" protocol, so use it when you feel like you're coming down with something, whenever you get off an airplane, and after contracting mysterious jungle illnesses brought on by powerful shamanic rituals.

Section 5. Jet Lag, Sleep, and Counting Sheep

Did you know that sleep deprivation is one of the gnarliest health issues plaguing American adults in our society?

Lack of sleep contributes to:

- Depression
- Skin aging
- Weight gain
- Less sex
- General unattractiveness
- More disagreements with your partner

Thirty-six percent of Americans also say they drive drowsy or have fallen asleep while driving. This is an unfortunately high number considering that going 17-19 hours without sleep is considered equivalent to having a blood-alcohol content (BAC) of .05.

Sleep deprivation is also linked to bigger waistlines. Sleeping less will increase your appetite because leptin (your appetite-regulating hormone) will decrease, causing feelings of hunger even if you don't need to eat.

Most people need to sleep 7 or more hours per night, but younger people need even more than that, and kids younger than 5 years of age need 10-12 hours every night!

Getting the right amount of sleep is crucial to your performance at work and your ability to adventure on vacation, as well as your overall health and vitality.

Even with all the scientific advancements over the years, doctors still don't fully understand sleep or why it's so important. All we know is that yes, it's a huge deal, and not getting enough sleep will make you a grouchier version of yourself.

What do you do when your best plans still don't allow you to get a full night of sleep? Restlessness, insomnia, and sleep apnea affect millions of Americans, and that doesn't even include jet lag. Many of my road-warrior clients complain about the effect that jet lag has on their energy and health in the first few days in any new location.

Even with the best intentions, jet lag can derail our progress, as well as our everyday function.

Tips from a Professional Traveler

During our year of travel we logged:

- 247 hours on buses
- 23 flights
- 42 cities
- 55 hostels
- 166 miles hiked
- 115 miles biked
- 138 miles kayaked
- 7 hospital visits
- 6 animal bites

... and I would still only say that I'm a recreational traveler at best.

So, I asked Captain Catherine Drury, a career airline pilot who has logged more than 25,000 hours of flight time, for her best tips to avoid the menace of JET LAG. As an avid hiker, yogi, and gymnast, Catherine has an extremely active lifestyle when she's not flying.

Having strategies to mitigate the effects of traveling cross-country is very important to her overall well-being.

Here are her top tips:

Adjust to the Time Zone Before Landing

"So many times, I hear people say that they could never fall asleep because it's only 7 p.m. in Phoenix/ Seattle, or wherever they're from. So what?

If you're in New York, it's 10 p.m., and it's been dark for several hours.

Adopt the time zone that you're in, and quit cross-checking it with where you came from. It can be your brain that's holding you back from falling asleep. Be where you are."

Your body is remarkably adaptable, and let's be honest, you're probably a little sleep-deprived anyways. Going to sleep at 7 p.m. might be just what the doctor ordered, and it's going to set you up for success in the following days.

This doesn't just apply to sleep habits. Captain Drury suggests that we adopt the time zone of wherever we're going before leaving. So, if you're flying somewhere that's 7 or more hours ahead, start adjusting your mind to the reality of that time zone before you even get on the plane.

While the time change across continents is difficult, the maximum of 3 hours' difference anywhere in the continental United States shouldn't have a large impact on your sleep or wake-up schedule.

Before leaving on your trip, adjust your mental clock to be in line with wherever you're going to end up.

Children of the Sun

The body's circadian rhythm is highly dependent on sunlight. In fact, when people lived in the dark without clocks for a month, their bodies adopted a 25-hour rhythm rather than 24.

I get it though: We often walk off the plane and into a conference room with no windows and artificial light for the rest of the day. But given the option to get outside on a break or when you first arrive, take some time to get some natural light and adjust physically to where you are.

Even if you can only get outside in the evening, that's OK, too. Being outside is important because it lets your body understand and adapt to where you are. If you take a walk at night, you'll naturally start calming down in preparation for hibernation.

Get Moving!

Sitting all day is a killer of motivation and disrupter of normal sleep patterns. But sometimes that's just what we have to do because it's not yet socially acceptable to knock out jump squats in the corner during an intense board meeting.

NATE'S HOT TIP

Walking burns fat better than many other forms of exercise, will help reset a cranky back through self-alignment, and can be helpful in boosting your immune system to combat colds and flus. Walking should be a part of your routine at home as well as on the road..

So, it's important that, when given the option, we take some time to get outside and walk around.

Let's just take a minute and appreciate how dope walking is.

The ability to walk long distances is one of the key mechanisms that has allowed humans to flourish and populate over our history, and we're engineered to be able to do it better than almost any other animal.

The way our muscles, bones, and joints work create harmony between the tissue to move in a forward motion. Walking is innate and automatic, and you should do it as often as possible.

It's also a great way to get grounded mentally, relieve stress, and help detox from a stressful day. Throw in some headphones with your favorite music or a podcast, and just wander.

Walking is important, especially if you don't really feel like making it to the gym on your first travel day. Any kind of movement will do wonders for your mood, your body, and your brain.

Working out can help clear brain fog that we get being in another time zone and traveling all day. If you're going to train on the first day you arrive, focus on the cardio elements of your training and lift weights in a higher rep range to sweat more and breathe hard.

A higher rep range is a better option because it keeps you from going too heavy after being stuck in a non-optimal position for most of the day. Training will also make your body more tired, which will help you sleep more soundly at night.

- Opt for timed sets of 40-60 seconds per exercise.
- Do 45 minutes and then get on with your life.
- Include single-leg and arm versions of your favorite exercises
- Do direct core work, but make sure you're doing a 2:1 ratio of "anti" core moves to crunch style moves.
- Avoid working out right before bed because that will wake up your body and make falling asleep more difficult.

Nap Ahead of Time

When Captain Drury goes on a red-eye flight, she tries to get a little bit of extra sleep ahead of time to make up for the fact that she's not allowed to catch a quick nap on the plane ... you know, being the one in charge and all.

By getting a 1-2-hour nap before the flight, she's fresher for work and doesn't experience the same negative impact on her sleep cycle.

Many of us plan to sleep on the flight, and for someone like my wife whose superpower is sleeping anywhere, that's great!

But if you know yourself, and that your sleep on an airplane will be fragmented and not enjoyable, try to grab a nap ahead of time and then spend some time reading on the plane. For best (sleepiest) results, try busting out that old anatomy textbook from college.

If reading about how the kidneys process toxins doesn't start to make those eyelids heavy, you might want to think about Nate's Super Sleep Solution (below).

Tips from a Recreational Traveler

Here are some of MY top tips for dealing with jet lag, falling asleep, and sleeping in crowded and smelly places. These are based purely on my experiences traveling thousands of miles in buses, trains, airplanes, and vans.

It should be noted that I'm not a doctor, and that this advice is purely anecdotal and not intended to treat, cure, or prevent any diseases.

How to Fall Asleep on an Airplane 100 Percent of the Time

If you're traveling for 6 or more hours, or overnight, but don't think you can fall asleep, here's what I do:

Let me reiterate, *I'm not a doctor, this is bad advice, don't do it.* That being said...

- Step 1. Take 1–2 Benadryl
- Step 2. Have a cocktail or tiny, airplane-sized bottle of wine
- Step 3. Drool on neighbor for 4 ½ hours.
- Step 4. Wake up after sleeping on your arms for hours. Your hands don't work, you can't talk well, opening your eyes is unpleasant at best. Your hands may never work again. It's impossible to open this stupid airplane dinner. Who invented plastic wrap? Why don't I have any control of my fingers? Don't look the flight attendant in the eye.
- Step 5. Put your hood back up and go to sleep for another 45 minutes.
- Step 6. You feel better ... ish. There's still a significant veil of brain fog.
- Step 7. Land. Walk around for 30 minutes. There it is! You feel like yourself again.

DON'T COUNT HOURS OF SLEEP

Here's a fun game that everyone plays with themselves. Stop me if you've heard this one before.

Set your alarm for 6 a.m.

Look at the time, it's 10:42 p.m. "That means if I fall asleep right now, I'll get 7 hours and 18 minutes of sleep."

But of course you don't fall asleep that minute. You lay in bed for a while thinking about the comeback you should have said to the bully in seventh grade, or preparing imaginary arguments with your significant other.

You wake up. "Ugh, I didn't get enough sleep last night"

STAHHHHP.

Seriously – this is a bad habit. Here's why.

1. When you wake up and immediately say "I didn't get enough ..." You start the day in with a feeling of scarcity. Of not having or being enough. This is a negative mindset, and it starts the day on a bad foot even if you don't realize it overtly.

Yeah, 7 or more hours of sleep is ideal, but if you didn't get it, too bad! You can't go back to sleep, you have work to do! Moping about it and spending time thinking about the sleep you didn't get is like being a

30-year-old stuck telling the same story about how your seventh-grade girlfriend broke up with you in sixth period after you asked her out at lunch the same day (But I'm not bitter Jessica Cirillo).

2. Placebo sleep. It's a big deal!

You've heard of the placebo effect, right? Basically, it means that people who take sugar pills they think help build muscle, cure yellow fever, or give them energy, will often end up with the result *THEY BELIEVED* would happen.

Same when it comes to sleep. If you wake up and think to yourself, *"Wow, I got a lot of good sleep last night,"* you'll feel BETTER than your counterparts who got the same amount of sleep but woke up and immediately started telling themselves about how tired they are.

Your brain is the biggest muscle in your body. The more you train it to behave the way you want it to, the better you'll be at these behaviors. Remember how we talked about "owning it" earlier? This is a great way to practice that mindset.

Inversions

Inversions come from yoga, and simply indicate any position that you're in where your head is below your heart. These little gems can be incredibly simple and effective at helping you get to sleep, and you don't need to be able to pull off any circus moves to make them effective.

The most important thing is finding a position that is comfortable and allows you to control your breathing. If you're stress-breathing, you'll be less relaxed than when you started.

Take deep breaths into the diaphragm or lower belly while holding these poses. Start with the easier options, but feel free to try the harder ones. Remember, this isn't about pushing yourself, just relaxing.

- Child's pose – Easy
  - ° Kneel on the floor or mat with your knees wide, but your big toes touching. Push your butt way back and try to rest it on your heels while your head goes forehead to the floor and your arms reach way out in front. Extend your arms, breathe deeply, and then focus on relaxing your body, starting with your hands and working down to your feet.

- Downward facing dog - Medium
  - ° Start in a pushup position with your hands and feet on the ground. Push your butt back as far as you can until you feel a stretch in the back of your legs. Try to keep your back flat, and keep your shoulders *away* from your ears. Relax, and breathe.

- Headstand – Advanced
  - You can go freestanding if you're brave, or if you've done it before, otherwise use a wall. Put your head closest to the wall, then place both hands on the ground farther from the wall so that your hands and head form a tripod to support your body.

    Jump or lift your legs up above your head (use the wall if you need to), and then extend your legs. Feel free to put your legs in different positions. Feet together, knees bent, both legs wide and extended – try different versions.

    Breathe, relax, and make sure that you're supporting at least two-thirds of the pressure with your hands rather than your head and neck.

READING

Like we talked about earlier, reading can be beneficial to make you tired. For proof of this, I just think back to my worst college classes. I never slept better than when I was "reading" my environmental psychology book that was written in 1952.

Not only was the content bone-dry, it was written in verbose flowery language that caused me to resent the author, the book, the class, and the school.

You don't have to pick up a textbook to make this work, but I'd stay away from exciting content and "page-turners" if you're using a book as a sleep aid. Psychology, business, and biographical books seem to work well for this.

I'd avoid "50 Shades of Grey" or the Twilight series. Not because of the sleep thing; just on principle.

BLACK OUT

You can black out through a variety of means, but I'm not talking about the type that comes after too many Four Lokos – rather the state of closing yourself off from the world.

We already addressed some of the most necessary items to pack on trips, but using a sleep mask and headphones/earplugs can be the difference between tranquility and anger as you listen to that baby cry a few rows away.

In a pinch, you can always use the hood of a sweatshirt or a beanie to cover your eyes, but the sleep mask is the most comfortable, plus people will always be remarking on how cool you look when you wear it.

Ear plugs are a good idea, but I really prefer headphones with some low-key music playing. Find a playlist you like, or make one up. I always prefer to put on something ambient with no words. Leo Kottke's

"6-String Guitar" albums are some of my favorite for relaxation.

SLEEP SUPPLEMENTS

Google "sleep supplements" and you'll get about 19 million results.

There are a lot of supplement companies that promise to help with sleeping, but few that deliver. Here's a list of supplements that have been proven to help you get more sleep, or a higher quality of sleep.

- Zinc
  - ° Zinc is a mineral with numerous health benefits. It supports a healthy immune system and healthy hormone levels in men and women, which is important for getting a good night's sleep.
- Magnesium
  - ° Magnesium is well known for its ability to relieve insomnia. One study found that it helps decrease cortisol, the "stress hormone" that can keep you up at night. It also helps muscles relax, to give you that calm "sleepy" feeling and to help you unwind after a long day.
- Melatonin
  - ° Melatonin is a naturally produced substance in the body that contributes to the circadian

rhythm and sleep cycles. Taking small doses of this supplement can help re-establish healthy sleep patterns, as well as give you some vivid dreams.

One time I could have sworn that I was surrounded by indigenous Indians in the rainforest who were all chanting "U-G-L-Y you ain't got no alibi. You ugly! You, you ugly!"

But I think that was more cause I was dared to eat a really brightly colored caterpillar — not just cause I took melatonin.

- GABA
  - ° Gamma-Aminobutyric Acid (GABA) is one of your body's primary neurotransmitters, and acts to calm your central nervous system (CNS). Research has shown the GABA supplement to be effective in natural treatment for depression, anxiety, insomnia, and addiction.

- 5-HTP
  - ° 5-Hydroxytryptophan (5-HTP) replenishes serotonin levels, providing new stores of this necessary neurotransmitter in the brain. Tryptophan supplements like 5-HTP have a long history of use for treating depression

and anxiety disorders, and for enhancing sleep.

BED-TIME ROUTINE FOR MAXIMUM SLEEPINESS

All of this is good information, but a little overwhelming in its scope.

Here's how to put it all together for a great night's sleep: We'll assume you're probably not tired but need to get up early to start your day off right.

1. Take a 30-minute walk after dinner. This will help you digest your food and start to relax.
2. When you get back to your room, put on some low-key music and make a cup of herbal tea.
3. Set the thermostat for 68-72 degrees if possible. It's easier to sleep in colder rooms.
4. Do 5-10 minutes of stretching and inversions. Focus on deep belly breathing and taking inventory of your body.
   a. This means starting at the top of your head, and slowly moving down, actively relaxing each part of your body as you go.
5. Take whatever sleep supplements you've been using.
6. Get in bed and grab a book. Now is the time to put your sleep mask on your forehead or earplugs in. These act as a trigger to signal to your body that

it's bed time. (They become more powerful the more often you use them.)

7. Read until you're feeling drowsy. Put the book up, turn the lights off, put the sleep mask on and the earplugs in.

8. Good night!

Section 6. Every Hotel Room Is A Gym

Sometimes luxurious and sometimes trashy, lodging is always a big part of traveling. We often have the autonomy to choose where we stay, but occasionally we don't.

Picking the right place to stay in the right area can be crucial to our success in maintaining our active lifestyle, but it's also important to remain flexible and mobile enough to work with less-than-ideal circumstances.

Traveling around the world with all my possessions strapped to my back, I found that the most ideal option was to bring a suspension strap that enabled me to do high-intensity exercise on the beach, in laundry rooms, on college campuses or in the heart of the jungle.

That way, when I found a hotel gym that was serviceable it was always a bonus, but I never counted on it. With the suspension strap, I was never without an excuse to get in a training session.

The #1 predictor of success is consistency. Not supplements, not fancy leggings, and not if you can afford a personal trainer.

That's why it's incredibly important to always have a way of getting in a quick and dirty workout – no matter where you wake up.

HOTELS

There are several hotels that have incorporated health and fitness into their brand, which sets them apart in the high-end hotel market. If you have the chance to stay at one of these chains, you'll be treated to services like a concierge that will bring gym clothes and shoes to your room, free gym memberships at high-end health clubs for the duration of your stay, or hotel gym workout classes.

Here are the best of the best:

WESTIN

Starwood's high-end hotel, the Westin will deliver shoes and clothes to your room, and their front desk staff will have mapped out the best 3- and 5-mile runs nearby.

They also offer exercise videos that you can do in the gym, and even routines that you can do on the floor.

Fairmont

The Fairmont hotels have teamed up with Reebok to deliver training equipment and clothes to your room for free.

Guests can have a yoga mat, an exercise band, an exercise shirt, shorts, and shoes dropped off for them so there's no excuse not to get a workout in.

The Standard

These hotels are in some of the largest centers of commerce in the U.S., and have partnered with Peloton bikes to give guest a spin class experience in the privacy of their high-end fitness centers.

Guests can choose from different instructors and types of classes when selecting a ride.

The Fairfield Inn and Suites

Marriott's high-end, lifestyle-based hotel chain. Guests can use the fitness center which has helpful videos and tips from Lifetime Fitness.

Guests who stay there are also able to use any of Lifetime Fitness' gyms for up to 7 days after their stay at the Fairfield.

How to Set Up Your Own Gym
ANYWHERE

Despite our best efforts and the amenities provided to us, sometimes the hotel gym just doesn't work for us. Either it closes as inopportune times, only has four old dumbbells for use, or is packed full of sweaty individuals from the conference you're attending.

However, the suggestions in the Hotel Section are great if you have the luxury of staying at whatever chain you want, or if your company will spring for you to stay at the Westin so long as you only get ONE facial per day. These are probably more likely if you fall into the category of "professional traveler." If you're traveling on a budget or prefer staying in Airbnbs rather than large chains, you'll find the following suggestions helpful.

Sometimes, turning your hotel room/patio/park/laundry-room-in-a-dirty-Colombian-hostel into a gym can be the best option, especially if you're only able to squeeze in a 15-30-minute workout.

Sometimes you work out because exercise is important. Other times you work out because it's therapy and the people you're with will hate you if you don't stop spazzing out and burn some energy.

We had been staying at Hostel Iguana in Santa Marta, Colombia. for a of couple days while recovering from a four-day jungle trek. After struggling through a couple chapters of "Chicken Soup for the Horse Lover's Soul" in Spanish (classic hostel reading), I needed a good workout because I get antsy without exercise.

The problem was that there were NO good doors to set up my suspension strap except the one that went in and out of hostel's laundry room. So, during a lull in the middle of the day, I set up my workout space and started cranking out a lower-body routine that had me burning, sweating, and crying (just a little).

It wasn't until I was halfway into the workout that I realized that all the employees of the business were eating lunch in a room directly to the side of where I had chosen to train. So, they had been watching my entire workout, including the time I stopped to scratch the gnarly butt itch that had been plaguing me since our long trek.

Good workouts are rarely glamourous, but always effective. This one had no charm whatsoever, but was exactly what I needed.

You only need two things to get a good workout:

- Some type of resistance (bodyweight, suitcase, bands)
- A good training program

The program is the most important piece. Not just having it in your hand, but also knowing how to use it effectively. You could have the world's best program, but if you pull it out for the very first time when you only have 15 minutes to train, you're not going to get an effective session.

RESISTANCE

Since you bring your body with you wherever you go, it's a great option that can be used for an effective workout without any other equipment at all.

I prefer to bring a suspension strap with me to ensure I can use my body in different ways and movement patterns, and because to be honest – pure bodyweight training can get boring.

That's why using a strap, bands, or sliders can not only provide you a more effective workout, it's also more fun. While a lot of us don't think of training as being fun, having new implements or exercises to do will also increase adherence to the program – which is what we need.

Your suitcase can also provide resistance, and can be used for a ton of different exercises. Hold it to your chest, put it on your shoulders, or lift it above your head.

These techniques can be quite effective in core training, or just making in-hotel training more interesting.

The downside is that the more organized you are with your packing and unpacking, the lighter your suitcase will be. You can always stuff random things from the hotel into the suitcase to add weight, but it's hard to explain to the manager why you were leaving with the hotel lamp in your suitcase.

Programming

Setting up your own ideal program is outside of the scope of this book, but I will tell you that the flow is important. Minimal time should be spent on transitioning between exercises, since we're assuming hotel-room workouts need to maximize a short amount of time.

Depending on personal fitness levels, I like to set up circuits of 2-4 exercises, alternating between body parts.

For example:

1. Suspension-strap bicep curl
2. Band triceps extension
3. Reverse lunge on slider

This way we can move through several exercises in a row without getting overly tired in a single muscle group. This provides a better training effect that will help you burn more calories and train harder in a short amount of time.

If you're using your suitcase, set up your program as "complexes." This just means to do a certain number of reps of one exercise before moving on to the next. Finish all the exercises without putting your suitcase down, and then rest.

For example:

1. Suitcase overhead presses
2. Suitcase lunge
3. Suitcase squat
4. Suitcase front raise

Do each exercise for 40 seconds, and rest 1 minute between rounds.

This is an effective training strategy if you only have one weight implement and want to do a convenient and high-intensity exercise session.

However, you decide to go about maximizing your space for a workout, make sure that you already have a training session written out or decided on before you start. It's easy to slack off if you're not sure what you're going to do next, and with a shorter session, like the one you'd do in a hotel, you need to be maximizing a short amount of time instead of relying on your brain to come up with new exercises mid-session. Standing on your bed naked, spinning your suitcase around your body while screaming is a *fine* exercise, but it comes with a high risk, especially if you've decided to cover your body in non-organic coconut oil.

I help my clients out by sending them programs for every day of the week using only equipment that they can pack in a carry-on bag.

Every workout is programmed to be between 15 and 35 minutes, and can be done in 4 square feet of space in a hotel room. The exercises link to videos to ensure that there's no confusion about what the form of each exercise looks like.

If you're the type of person who is already prioritizing your health enough to be working out when your friends and colleagues are sleeping, then the rest of the process should be as easy as possible for you.

Bod in a Box

If you're looking for an easy-to-transport, totally inclusive fitness system, I created a product called <u>Bod in a Box</u> that is ideal for anyone who travels for work or pleasure and wants to ensure that they can get a great workout no matter where they're at.

Bod in a Box contains a suspension strap, two 40-inch bands (1/2-inch and 1-inch), and core sliders, all of which fit easily into a carry-on bag or backpack.

Bod in a Box also comes with a monthly program that gets harder as you get stronger. You can get more information at bodinabox.com

Section 7. Morning Ritual

The first 30 minutes within waking up are the most important part of your day.

This block of time sets the tone for the rest of your day and can go a long way toward helping you be productive and get the most out of your time.

Alternately, you can scroll through Instagram and see what everyone else was up to while you were sleeping.

If you're a motivated person with goals to hit, you need to take advantage of this time, and set yourself up for success in your day by having a morning routine.

In the past few years, much research has been done on the importance of utilizing the first waking moments of your day to increase productivity, energy, and a positive mindset. Since we're developing habits that will help us stay fit and healthy while traveling, the first 30 minutes can make or break the day.

A lot of people that I respect have put together great morning routines. Among them:

Hal Elrod, author of "The Miracle Morning," uses an acronym called **SAVERS** in his daily routine. This stands for Silence, Affirmations, Visualization, Exercise, Reading, and Scribing. More from Hal at HalElrod.com

Mark Sisson, the founder of The Primal Blueprint, takes a cold dip in the pool, does some balance exercises, and then does a crossword puzzle while waiting for his coffee. You can find more from Mark at MarksDailyApple.com

Most successful people have some morning routine, and they always include some aspect of exercise, mindfulness, and coffee.

Your morning ritual will evolve and change over time as you find things that you prefer, but it's important to have some sort of pattern to the beginning of the day. Mine has evolved into what it is today through a variety of influences, and finding what works for me, but you can take from this as you see fit for your life.

Even if your morning ritual looks different from these, consistency in positive habits is key.

The Morning Domin8tion Rituals are fairly intense, but have calmed down quite a bit after I eliminated the morning ritual–blood sacrifice.

MORNING DOMIN8ION RITUALS — NOT FOR THE FAINT OF HEART

1. WTFU —Don't Hit the Snooze Button
2. HYDRATE! - Drink 24-32 ounces of water
3. TRAIN — Get in your workout early.
4. THE FLINCH — Get in the shower while it's cold.
5. HEALTH INSURANCE — take Vitamin D, fish oil, antioxidants.
6. BRAIN — Read 5 minutes from a motivational book of your choice.

WTFU

Hitting the snooze on your alarm is a bad choice because it doesn't greet the day with energy and vitality. Your first thought of the day is super important, and if that thought is, "Oh shit, it's already morning," you're starting off on the wrong note.

When your alarm goes off, your first thought should be "YES!" (Mine is normally, "YES! COFFEE!!") Even if you didn't sleep well, remember: Focusing on *how good* you feel can improve your day.

Set your phone away from your bed to require yourself to get up to turn it off. Or request a wakeup call (or two) at your hotel.

HYDRATE

We dehydrate ourselves all night by breathing out our moist air *(Side note: Did you remember that's how we lose fat? By breathing it out?)*

Dehydration can sap your energy and strength. A 3 percent decrease in hydration can cause up to 30 percent loss of power in the gym. That's the difference between benching 200 and 140.

Grab a big glass of room-temperature water and put it inside you before you put anything else in your body. Believe it or not, this will invigorate you more than slamming a cup of coffee... Plus, having the water first will give the coffee a more stimulating effect.

TRAIN

When we sharpen our bodies, our brains follow suit. Training in the morning is one of the best things you can do to ensure you have a successful and energetic day.

Plus, if you're looking for life-long results, you simply can't rely on nighttime workouts. They're too variable for many of us, and most of the time that's the time we're putting out fires at home or work, and we often have burned out our motivation muscle by the end of the day.

Even a 15-minute workout can elevate your mood and energy, but I prefer to spend 30 minutes each morning doing some sort of physical activity.

Doing heavy weights isn't recommended within an hour of waking up, so that's why I encourage people to do bodyweight training in the morning. Build strength, burn fat, and create a lean, muscular physique by mastering your own weight.

THE FLINCH

This is the part of the day where you decide that you're the boss and in charge of whatever happens to you. Turn your shower on cold, stare that bitch in the face, then get in. WOOOOOOO!

Aside from the physical benefits of cold-immersion therapy (decreased inflammation, increased blood flow, increased circulation, CNS stimulation, increased skin tightness), you'll also receive the mental benefit of facing an uncomfortable situation and confronting it.

This simple step can take your brain to the next level.

When you face a situation that you really don't want to be in, and still take the step to confront it, you reinforce the fact that you're a badass who does what they want, when they want, regardless of how you're *feeling* at the time.

79

HEALTH INSURANCE

Vitamin D and Omega-3 (fish oil) are both necessary on a daily basis. If you have a green supplement, antioxidants, or multivitamins, take those as well. See the *Supplements* section for my recommendations.

Vitamin D deficiency is so common now that doctors don't even check for it. They just assume everyone has it. Vitamin D is more of a hormone than a vitamin and helps with a ton of vital functions, including heart, skin, eyes, hair, bones, overall energy, and if that wasn't enough – body fat mobilization.

Take 2-5 drops per day. The drops absorb better than the capsules. You can find them at a health food store or on amazon.

Fish oil also can help decrease inflammation, belly fat, and help your joints feel better. Take 2 capsules of high-quality fish oil 1-2 times per day.

BRAIN

People often say that motivation doesn't last. Well, neither does bathing, which is why we recommend it daily. – Zig Ziglar

By starting the day focused, alert, and with something positive in our minds, we make it possible for every day to be as GREAT as possible.

Read a chapter from a book or listen to a podcast that fires you up. My two favorites are "The Greatest

Salesman in the World," by Zig Ziglar, and "Go for No," by Richard Fenton.

Pull from the Morning Domin8ion Routine when creating your own morning ritual. You might find that you need one morning routine for the time when you're home, and another one for when you're on the road.

I find that I prefer having an express option for when I'm running behind or have an early morning planned. Otherwise I do some variation of the morning domin8ion every day.

SECTION 8: EATING

Eating is a part of life, and has been for a long time. Several years in fact. The practice of eating goes back for at least 20 years before I was born – and before that, historians believe our ancient ancestors also engaged in mastication of plants and animals for sustenance.

I wasn't there, so I can't be sure.

What I do know is that eating and proper nutrition is one of the biggest hurdles for many people to stay in great physical condition year-round.

Many of us can work out 4-6 times per week religiously while drinking enough water and getting plenty of sleep, but we're plagued by the desire to eat TOO MUCH ice cream.

This compounds when we're traveling. Now we're out of our sphere of influence and don't have access to all the healthy snacks and meals we normally have at home. Plus, people want to take us to dinner and stuff us full of high-calorie food and drink.

Just closed a new deal? Better drink six glasses of wine and have two desserts then.

Just arrived in Philadelphia? Prolly should stop for a cheesesteak at 1 a.m.

Stuck in an airport with hungry co-workers? Skip the salad, let's all get Cinnabon.

You've probably heard that getting in shape is 80 percent nutrition and 20 percent exercise. Or perhaps you've seen your favorite Instagram celebrity touting that, "Abs are made in the kitchen," while they sip a "fat-burning" tea in their underwear.

I don't know about those percentages, and I've tried to build abs in the kitchen (the countertop is a terrible place for crunches). But what I do know is that it takes a consistent focus on not just eating less, but eating nourishing, nutritious foods at least 80% percent of the time to get and stay in good shape.

Yes, you should still be able to enjoy a slice of pie or a beer with friends, but really the only rule is that over the next year, 80 percent of your meals should be healthy, nutritious meals that feed your body and your brain.

If you can adhere to that one principle, you're farther ahead than most people in the world who bounce from diet to diet looking for a 6-week fix to undo their last 6 years of bad habits.

You're the result of your last 27,000 meals. No cleanse, pill, or powder is going to change that.

That said, I'm going to provide you with some easy, actionable ways to make eating healthy foods easier from a mental and time perspective. There isn't one diet that I think everyone should do or follow. Dogmatic thinking like that further confuses the issue, and makes it harder to find the truth about nutrition for those of us looking for a simple solution.

WHY DIETS WORK

Visit any book store in the U.S. and you'll find hundreds of books on diets and nutrition. Some promote healthy habits, while some advertise a more extreme approach.

Here are some of my favorite real diets:

Eating for Your Astrological Sign – Learn 10 reasons Leos should only eat animals off the endangered species list.

The Avoiding Swamps Diet – Have you ever noticed that bloated swampy feeling you get in Louisiana? Me either.

The Cotton Ball Diet – If you're hungry, just pop a zero-calorie cotton ball! It's a little dry, but the flavor is … dry. Super dry.

The Tongue Patch Diet – It's harder to eat if someone sews a big, painful patch on your tongue!

The Cigarette Diet – popularized by *actual* doctors in the 20s, this diet encourages smoking cigarettes instead of eating. That's good-quality health care.

Yes. These are all ridiculous and there's a 50 percent chance that you'll die if you try them, but here's the crazy thing though. All diets work.

Despite the differences that many of them tout, balancing hormones through intermittent fasting, using fat for fuel like the Ketogenic Diet, or eating pizza and ice cream using the "If It Fits Your Macros" approach, all diets will work by *creating a caloric deficit.*

No matter what the claim of the latest and greatest new diet, the results that people see are due to eating less food than the calories they're expending for energy.

For proof that all diets work through calorie restriction, look at Mark Haub. He tried to prove the opposite by going on a junk-food diet, but carefully monitoring his calories.

Haub is a nutrition professor at Kansas State University. And after countless discussions with students over "quality vs quantity," he went on a diet of Twinkies, candy bars, and powdered donuts for months, with the intent to see what his body did.

Haub ate only 1,800 calories per day. At the end of 2 months, he had lost 27 pounds only eating foods he found at convenience stores.

No, I'm not saying that is a good diet.

Yes, he probably felt pretty crummy the whole time.

And no, 1,800 calories of junk food isn't that much food. (One package of Hostess Mini Powdered Donuts is 1,100 calories.)

But the point is that diets work through creating a caloric deficit, not through the magic of eliminating one certain food group, or only eating carrots at midnight.

NATE'S HOT TIP

FOOD CHART

During the next few chapters I'll be talking about different foods as being proteins, carbs and fats. Here's the cheater guide to which foods fall into each category.

Carbohydrates: ALL VEGGIES, fruits, potatoes, sweet potatoes, rice, oatmeal, barley, quinoa, squash Necessary for energy, brain function, and high-intensity activities

Fats: Wild salmon, nuts, avocado, healthy oils (olive, avocado, coconut) Fuel for low-intensity activity like walking, as well as hormone function and overall health

Protein: Grass-fed beef, free-range chicken, eggs, wild fish, Greek yogurt, kefir Builds muscle and aids in recovery

What to Eat

So now that we know that there's no one perfect diet that will cause you to grow abs and star in a reality TV show, let's talk about what you should be eating.

The very simple explanation that everyone hates is this: Eat whole, real foods 80 percent of the time.

If your diet is basically the "ingredients" that make up other foods, you're doing it right.

While traveling through much of Central and South America, the problem I kept running into was a lack of fruits and veggies. Even though there's a large agricultural industry in many of those countries due to great growing conditions, most of the food available to order was brown.

Fried foods were the norm, and even when it wasn't fried, the diet was still mostly carbs. One meal I remember in particular was an appetizer of wheat soup with pork fat, a main dish of rice, chicken, French fries, and bread, with a glass of lemonade.

(Based on my experience, French Fries are the most popular food in the world)

However, it was still possible to eat well, it just required a little bit more work to search out markets where we could buy avocados, papayas, and my favorite, meat-on-a-stick.

One of my favorite meals was served from a cart on the side of the road where a guy was grilling chicken hearts, and we were cutting and eating a papaya that we had bought from another street vendor. It was simple, delicious (chicken hearts are surprisingly good, and full of protein), and neither of us got E. coli!

Choosing to eat ingredients rather than processed foods that come in boxes and bags is always the best option. Many diets fall back on this simple piece of advice, but give it different names, and apply slightly different rules. The most prevalent of which are the Paleo Diet, and the Whole 30 Diet.

These approaches take slightly dissimilar approaches to carbs and oils, but for the most part they are intended to be a return to eating foods that grow in the ground or were one time alive.

Eating this way has been proven to lower insulin resistance, help maintain lower blood sugar, reduce prevalence of heart disease, and help to maintain a healthy weight.

Without getting super sciency and talking about how leptin levels affect obesity and atherosclerosis, the ideal diet is whole foods that come in a full range of colors.

Your diet should be aimed at helping you feel and look your best, and while it's possible to lose fat while sipping Diet Cokes and eating low-fat Triscuits, you won't feel great, and you'll never look your best.

WHEN TO EAT

Although not as important as what to eat, meal timing is an important aspect of making your diet fit your lifestyle. If you're constantly trying to take a stringent approach while you're on the road and eat small servings of tilapia and rice, you're going to have a bad time.

In fact, let me just come out and say it. Eating 6 times per day is dumb. It's difficult and mind-numbing. Plus, toting Tupperware to your grandma's Christmas dinner doesn't make you a fitness model, it makes you a dweeb. And it's totally unreasonable when you're in and out of meetings all day long.

Studies show that eating 8 times per day is no different than eating 2 times per day if the overall calories and macronutrients are the same. Additionally, eating that often means that you're constantly digesting, and your body rarely enters *autophagy*, our natural detoxification process.

I prefer a carb-cycling approach, which means adjusting number of carbs eaten depending on activity for the day. On days without exercise, less carbs are required.

On hard workouts (read: leg days), eat more carbs post-workout to help with recovery.

Carb Cycling — Use it to Your Advantage on the Road

Carb cycling is one of the easiest ways to ensure that you're eating to your goals and energy requirements, while using a bio-hack to shuttle more of your calories to muscle and less to fat.

This works because your muscles need fuel after a workout, so eating some simple carbs from rice/oats/fruit is a great way to increase your insulin, which helps in transporting more nutrients to your hungry muscle cells.

Carb cycling is a great approach because it works with the body's natural processes, and it can be used with any diet you prefer.

Carb cycling requires at least a basic idea of where and what you're going to be eating throughout the day, and I've found it works better in conjunction with an earlier workout.

To use carb cycling, make sure to eat the majority of your carbs for the day within an hour on either side of your workout. An hour before your workout, enjoy a piece of fruit, oatmeal, or a small meal of chicken and

NATE'S HOT TIP

Some people prefer to work out on an empty stomach. There's really no benefit or detriment to that – it's all about what you prefer. If you're working out early, you might want a small amount of Greek yogurt, or a small protein shake before you start, but there are no magic fat-burning benefits to fasted cardio.

rice. The larger the pre-workout meal, the longer you should wait before training.

After the workout, have some fruit with your protein shake, rice, beans or even bread (if you don't have better options). Ensure that you are getting enough protein to help your muscles recover from the workout. Carb cycling increases blood sugar, which raises insulin, which is instrumental in shuttling nutrients to hungry muscle cells, so it's important to have protein in your system to refuel.

How to Eat for All-Day Energy on the Road

Everyone has likely tried multiple diet styles, modalities, or meal-timing practices. There are thousands of different diets put out by "experts," and books about weight loss line the shelves at the bookstore like bad wallpaper at your grandma's house.

While most of these diets speak to weight loss, a concept that 84 percent of Americans have dealt with at some point, most diet plans don't deal with the true nature of food – to give you energy.

By demonizing food and talking in terms of clean versus dirty, health food versus fast food, and organic, gluten-free vegan-friendly versus Panda Express, we've all but forgotten what food is supposed to do.

A 3-STEP APPROACH TO EATING

I brought three proven concepts together into one plan that takes food choices, nutrient timing, and hormones into account. This approach works with your body's natural rhythm and chemistry to ensure you won't be pounding coffee at 2 p.m. just to get through the day. By working *with* your body instead of against it, you can be effortlessly focused both at your job and the gym, with no pre-workout required.

By using these tactics, we're working with your body's normal functions intelligently to feel awake, think clearly, and sleep hard:

1. Carb Cycling: By eating most of your carbs after your workout, you'll never get the crash associated with spiking your blood sugar. This will also ensure your sleep is deeper and comes more effortlessly, in addition to making sure your muscles have all the fuel they need to develop and recover.

2. Nutrient Timing: By eating light for most of the day, your sympathetic nervous system stays active. This allows you to stay in fight-or-flight mode (or work-rapidly-on-your-spreadsheet mode).

Even though this evolutionary mechanism was intended to help humans stay alert while hunting, you can harness the power of this hunger and apply it when you need to focus and be productive. In contrast, getting stuffed on a big meal switches on your parasympathetic nervous system, which is designed for rest and relaxation, so your energy goes toward digestion.

If you want to be productive during the day, leverage your evolution and stay a *little* hungry.

3. Hormonal Balance: Our bodies are the site of countless chemical reactions that happen whether we want them to or are even aware of them. These reactions are normal hormonal responses to internal and external stimuli.

For example, cortisol is a stress hormone that gets a bad rep for increasing belly fat, but it also plays a role in energy production. Cortisol spikes in the morning soon after rising, and decreases about an hour later. By taking this into account, we can choose to have caffeine about an hour after rising instead of rolling out of bed and immediately pounding a latte.

That way, we can get the maximum energizing effect from the coffee. This plan works *with* your body's natural hormonal responses instead of against them to maximize energy and alertness during the day.

Morning

The first thing you should consume after waking is 24-32 ounces of water. Add a bit of lemon and apple cider vinegar for maximum benefit, but properly hydrating yourself is one of the best ways to stay energized and feeling good all day. This doesn't cost anything or require any fancy supplements.

While you drink your water, spend a few minutes doing some arm circles, neck circles, stretching your legs, and just moving. This will energize you more than your traditional cup of coffee and a cigarette.

For breakfast, make a protein shake. If you train in the evenings, use mostly proteins and fats. Use peanut butter (or PB2 for fewer calories), avocado, or full-fat Greek yogurt as a healthy fat. Use a scoop or two of protein and almond milk or water.

If you train in the morning, have a shake with proteins and carbs. Use a piece of fruit, or a meal-replacement shake that has between 10-30 grams of carbohydrates.

Try to keep your breakfast shake between 300-500 calories.

If you are a coffee or tea drinker, have your first cup 1 hour after you wake up. Because cortisol levels spike after waking, you get a 30-60-minute energy boost, and then dip after that. Drink coffee in conjunction with this dip in cortisol to get the most out of the caffeine.

AM: Proteins + Fats (+ Veggies!):

- Eggs and bacon/sausage on a bed of spinach.
- Protein shake with protein powder, peanut butter, almond milk, handful of spinach

SNACK

If you're a snacker, or if you get hungry before lunchtime, another protein-and-fat meal with a small amount of carbs is great.

AM or PM Snack:

- One apple and ½ cup of almonds
- Protein shake with protein and almond butter

LUNCH

Avoid the lunchtime carb binge and avoid eating heavy foods. I like to have a protein source along with a salad or piece of fruit. Chicken salad and an apple is a good option, or anything along those lines. This is an easy thing to get while eating out, and an easy thing to pack for lunch, so there's little excuse for having a bacon burger.

This sort of lunch will ensure you have plenty of energy to finish out the workday, and with a light meal in your stomach you won't be reduced into an afternoon zombie. Not to mention, science tells us that being in a zombie state will reduce your willpower if someone does happen to offer you the leftover donuts in the break room and will reduce your abilities to fight actual zombies if the need arises.

Lunch: Proteins + Fats + Veggies:

- Chicken salad and a pickle
- Taco salad

Pre- and Post-Workout

Your pre- and post-workout meals should be roughly the same from a macronutrient point of view – high in carbs (for energy), and high in protein (for recovery). You can use the Greek yogurt snack from above. Use a low- or non-fat Greek yogurt with double the berries or some added bananas or pineapple.

Pre-Workout: Proteins + Fruit:

- Plain Greek yogurt with berries
- Protein shake with protein powder, almond milk and half a banana

97

Post-Workout: Proteins + Starchy Carbs/Fruits:

- Protein shake with protein powder, fruit, almond milk
- Teriyaki chicken and rice
- Baked potato with pulled pork
- Oatmeal with fruit, almond milk, and protein powder

DINNER

Since you've now had a successful day and a great workout as well, dinner can be a larger meal. This is for a couple of reasons:

Eating a meal slightly higher in protein and carbs will aid in recovery from your workout.

Carbs will make you sleepy since your body has to use more resources for its digestion, so it's a nice, natural sleep aid in the form of your dinner.

I like to eat a starchy carb like white potatoes, sweet potatoes, rice, quinoa, or occasionally pasta. Have a protein source like chicken, fish, or steak, along with a veggie. Roasted veggies are tastier than any other way of cooking vegetables. That's a PSA for those of you who think that you must boil or steam veggies.

NATE'S HOT TIP

If you're looking to lose fat, keep the fruit and ditch the starch in your post-workout meal.

Dinner: Protein + Carb + Veggies:

- Crock Pot beef stew with potatoes
- BBQ chicken tacos with salsa
- Pulled pork with rice and veggies

Eating Out

Going out to eat is a great part of life. Having someone else cook food, bring it to you, and then clean up after you and your whole sloppy family is amazing!

It doesn't matter how much margarita you spill on the tablecloth, how many French fries your toddler throws on the ground, or how many Diet Coke refills your Aunt Ruth wants – someone else has to deal with your shit.

If you're part of the 91 percent of Americans who went to a sit-down restaurant in 2016, then congratulations. Not everyone gets to eat out, and truly appreciating that it's a privilege and a treat goes a long way toward a healthy lifestyle. But, 100 percent of my clients over the past 10 years have cited eating out as a major hindrance in pursuing their goal weight.

Eating out is unavoidable when you're traveling, and especially if you're on a business trip that has a couple of client dinners built in. But you can leverage some of the good habits you've built at home to keep from being derailed simply because your clients *had* to order a bloomin' onion at Outback Steakhouse.

It's difficult for many people to stick to a healthy plan when going out to eat, but this is easily remedied with some simple planning and a couple of guidelines.

There are many people who go out to eat without losing ground. People who have a health-conscious mindset and understand the whole picture of fueling their body have no trouble making ideal choices when they're at a restaurant.

No matter if you're at a client dinner, a work buffet, or simply out with the family on your yearly vacation to Orlando, use these simple rules to make a good choice when it comes to your dinner selection.

1. Protein-Centric

The first key to picking a good meal that will move you toward your goals instead of sending you into a fiery nosedive that culminates in a week-long Cinnabon binge is to choose a dish that's high in protein.

Normally this is going to a dish based around meat, but eggs or quinoa work as well. So you can instantly eliminate dishes like spaghetti and pizza. Every meal that your favorite ripped celebrity eats is centered around protein.

Sorry, lean people don't put pizza on their "frequently consumed" list. Get over it.

Protein is filling, hard to convert to fat, and great for refueling and building muscle. It's very difficult to consume enough to cause liver or kidney problems, especially if you're drinking enough water. Besides, eating too much chicken is not your problem.

Rule: Make protein the focal point of your meal.

2. The Drinking Donut
Don't drink while you eat. Period.

Beer and health goals go together like my Uncle Luke and not marrying a hooker in Vegas. We'll talk more about alcohol later, but since alcohol is a poison, when you drink it, it sends your body into panic mode and shuts down all other processes besides priority Alpha: *getting this alcohol out of my body.*

If you drink, avoid snacking for an hour after you finish drinking. After eating, wait at least an hour to resume imbibing.

Rule: Don't drink and eat at the same time, wait an hour between.

3. Crème Fraiche
One way restaurants can make your food more delicious and artery-clogging is by adding more

101

oils and creams to things that you might not think need to be soaked in alfredo sauce or vegetable oil.

The best way to avoid this is by n*ot ordering food that includes a "cream sauce."*

Or – get this – since you're at a restaurant, you *could* tell the waiter to put your sauce on the side, or in the trash! You could also order your food precut and served in 27 butter dishes also, but, fun surprise, one will be filled with human spit.

Rule: Avoid cream sauces.

4. Freedom Fries

On the count of three, let's both say a food that isn't good for staying healthy, strong, or lean.

Too late! It's French fries. Even though bottomless fries come with literally every dish on the Red Robin menu, that doesn't mean you have to eat them all to get your money's worth.

Ninety-nine percent of restaurants will let you swap your fries for a non-artery clogging option. And the 1 percent? Those are the restaurants that your parents told you that you'd work if you didn't study.

Rule: Avoid French fries and deep-fried foods.

5. Carbs = Energy

After you pick what protein you want, pick your carbs based on your activity level for the day.

Seated at work + a workout with goal of fat loss = Just veggies

Seated at work + a workout with a goal of muscle gain = Single palm-sized serving of natural carbs (potato, rice, quinoa, beans)

Active at work + workout = Two palm-sized servings of natural carbs

Rule: Pick your carbs based on your activity (... and French fries aren't carbs).

6. Check Yourself

Pull up the menu before you get to the restaurant to avoid making a bad choice, especially if you haven't eaten in a few hours. Being tired or hungry (or intoxicated) can lead to worse food choices, so having a clear order before you get to the restaurant is a great way to make sure you are opting for the healthiest choice.

Rule: Check the menu before you get to the restaurant.

7. You're the Boss, Bitch.

If you go to a restaurant and literally don't see anything healthy on the menu, or if the menu is written on a chalkboard in German during every new moon – don't be afraid to ask the waiter.

Most restaurants will serve you a chicken breast and some mixed veggies if you say please. Many people think that since they're at a Chinese restaurant, they *must* order the deep-fried orange chicken. Hot tip: You don't.

Going to restaurants is a nice treat that we should be thankful for, but it's not an excuse for indulgence.

Rule: Ask the waiter for a grilled chicken breast and veggies.

Don't forget ...

It's OK to skip a meal. Your body can go 70 hours without food before you lose even one speck of your hard-earned muscle. (And just FYI, you can go for 10-plus days before you die.)

Skipping a meal isn't a death sentence, and feeling a little bit of hunger is fine. It's called "being human." Just because Americans haven't felt hungry since the mid-1930s doesn't mean that it's a bad thing.

CLIENT DINNERS

We're all born, we all die, and somewhere in the middle we all have to go to dinner with a client.

So how do you navigate a menu and make healthy choices but still have a good time eating and enjoying delicious food?

Here's what to do when you know you're headed out for a dinner on someone else's dime.

1. Eat Light
Since you're probably trying to impress someone, avoid a heavy meal of nachos or wings. Although they are delicious, eating sticky finger foods makes you look messy and unprofessional, in addition to not doing much for your waistline.

Ditch super-chewy foods like steaks. There's nothing worse than trying to frantically chomp through a filet when asked a question. Avoid the embarrassment and potential choking hazard by picking something that's light and easy to eat. (Remember to check the menu beforehand so you already know what you're gonna order.)

Rule: Pick a light meal that isn't messy or chewy.

2. Crush Water – Step away from the sodas and iced teas, water is your abs best friend.

You often can't control that your client just bought four bottles of wine for the price of your kid's college tuition, but you can adhere to the drinking donut we talked about earlier. Even in situations where you are having a glass of wine with dinner, it's still important to prioritize water.

Nothing worse than getting hammered at a client dinner and having to make an apology phone call while still slightly drunk the next morning.

Try to get at least one glass of water for every glass of *anything else* you drink that night. Having a big glass of water before you go to dinner is also helpful in managing cravings. Our stomachs respond to volume of food, not calories, so filling up slightly before going out to an indulgent restaurant is helpful in managing hunger when you see that they have all four of your favorite types of cheesecake.

Rule: One glass of water between every other drink you have.

3. Cheat-Day Mentality

We often get into the thought process that since we're only going to be in Houston once, we should take advantage of that and eat and drink until we're sick. That's a big bummer, because Houston is ... well, fine, but habitually using that logic results in needing new pants.

However, if you can get in the habit of training every day, you'll have built in some caloric insurance through the calories burned during exercise, and the "afterburn" effect that daily workouts have on your metabolism.

If you know that there is going to be a lavish client dinner in your future that you've been looking forward to all year, preload your day with a heavy-duty workout focusing on the full body and biggest muscle groups.

Don't neglect the quads and glutes, the two biggest muscles in the body. Training hard and then eating a bigger-than-average meal can be beneficial for building muscle, IF it's not an everyday habit.

Using meals like this to "shock" your system with higher calories is beneficial to being leaner and more muscular because it doesn't allow your metabolism to adapt to a standard caloric intake.

For best results, do an intense workout within 12 hours (although 3 hours is ideal).

Rule: If you're gonna eat big, make sure to get a good workout beforehand.

4. Savor the Flavor

Going out, especially to nice restaurants, shouldn't be all calorie counting and nervously avoiding wine. Take the time to try something new, and really enjoy eating your food.

This advice applies all the time, but honestly if you're out at Chili's for a work lunch – calm down Dave, it's nothing you haven't had before. Why don't you just go with the salad?

Eat slower than you normally would, and spend more time chewing and enjoying the flavors of your food.

If it's helpful to remember that many people around the world don't get to eat delicious food that is prepared for them by professional chefs – do that.

Rule: Slow down and chew your food for twice as long as you normally would.

5. Avoid Alcohol

Yeah, I know this one is hard, especially when you know the next stop is a karaoke bar, and you'll probably get asked to sing *Unbreak My Heart* by the illustrious Toni Braxton, again ... but remember that combining alcohol and food is a great precursor for wearing jeans with elastic in them.

If you're going to drink, have a meal with primarily proteins and fats 1-2 hours beforehand, and limit all calories after that. That means no beer, wine, or soda mixers.

Stick to clear alcohol with calorie-free mixers like soda water. Add a couple of limes for flavor. Getting drunk isn't about how your drink tastes, it's about the percentage chance you have of getting on the bar and having to send out apology emails the next day.

Rule: Stop drinking an hour before you eat, and don't drink within an hour of eating.

FAST FOOD

You're a real person. As awesome as it would be to have all your meals prepped for the week in perfect Tupperware in your perfect kitchen, with your perfect family, and perfect designer dog, life can often get in the way.

Tell me if this sounds familiar.

You wake up in a hotel in an unfamiliar city with 90 minutes before you must be in meetings for 10-12 hours (if you're lucky). You grab a quick bite to eat at the continental breakfast before hustling out the door to try to find your client's office. An hour and a half later, you're hungry again, with nothing to eat except strip-mall food or Wendy's. Oh well, there goes the diet.

We all want to be healthy and make good choices, but it's hard when life has other designs on your time. And going without food for most of the day inevitably leads to a massive binge when you finally encounter food, like a bear coming out of hibernation.

At some point, you give in and park yourself in the drive through. "Diet starts tomorrow," you think, as you shame-eat a cheesy-beef burrito in 2 bites.

What are you gonna do when your plans change, and you find yourself stuck in the food court at the airport for another 3 hours, or have to pick up a quick bite on the way to work because it's hard to fake a convincing smile when you're dead hungry?

What to Order at Fast Food Restaurants

If you follow the same rules as you do when going out to eat, you'll be on the right track, but there's another simple and effective solution:

Just order chicken salad or wraps.

It's a simple rule, but most pieces of extremely effective advice are.

Of course, there are other options of things to eat when you go out, but that goes beyond the scope of this book. To learn more, go to https://n8trainingsystems.

com/get-ripped-eating-fast-food-healthy-fast-food/ and download my guide to "Get Ripped Eating Fast Food."

It's a handy guide that will show you the three best meals at the 15 most popular and prevalent fast food chains in the world.

What to Never Order at a Fast Food Restaurant

If you head out the door and drop in at the food court but don't have this handy guide with you, avoid these gut busters.

Fried Food – Obvious, right? No matter how much you like them, French fries aren't getting you any closer to your body goals, nor will they help you feel alert and energized in 2 hours.

French fries in the U.S. are engineered by sadistic employees of Big Pharma (or maybe the illuminati, need more research) to provide the maximum amount of taste pleasure and the minimum amount of chewing, resulting in a deep, primal urge to shovel them into our faces as fast as we can.

They're fried perfectly, coated in a light topping of oil and sugar, and then rolled in salt. A perfect food designed to hit all the pleasure receptors of the brain.

If you can help it, also try to avoid ordering chicken or fish that's been fried, as many restaurants offer a grilled option of the same type of meal.

Drinks – Another no-brainer. Soda, sweet tea, and even fruit juices are often made with high fructose corn syrup and are high in calories and sugar. Ditching the drinks is an easy way to avoid several hundred calories, and avoid spending an additional 2 bucks. You're welcome!

Sauces – I know, I know. I love *all* sauces. The problem is that most sauces have a ton of sugar (ketchup, I'm looking at you). A sweet chili sauce can have as much as 8g of sugar per tablespoon, and I NEVER use just one tablespoon.

When ordering sandwiches or wraps, always ask for no mayo or ranch. Creamy dressings have a ton of fat in them and can add a couple-hundred unhealthy calories to what could have been a good meal.

Honorable mentions though are hot sauce (0 calories) and mustard (between 0-10 calories). But not honey mustard! I see you thinking it. Don't try.

NATE'S HOT TIP

Actual question people ask me: Is diet soda good for you?

Obvious answer: No. No it's not.

It's a chemical-laden diuretic that will dehydrate you, sneak into your house, and go through your underwear drawer. Just get water.

Alcohol

We've all been to the awkward work event where Gerald from Sales is stumbling through a monologue about "those people" while your creepy client from Omaha with the pornstache is close-talking to you about all the places he's been in his RV, and it seems like the only reasonable solution is to get very, very drunk.

T-minus 37 minutes until I need to take off my pants and play "Bang, Marry, Kill" with colleagues. What do you mean it's only Tuesday?

Alcohol is a part of our culture. Friday Happy Hour calls for buckets of beers, closing a big sale means your company is springing for champagne, and on Cinco de Mayo we honor our world heritage by drinking too much tequila and puking in our purses.

Now, if you wanted to live a life of puritanical restriction and stay lean, healthy, and feel good most of the time, you would give up alcohol completely.

Yea, I know you've seen the magazine covers and tabloids that read: "Glass of wine = 20-minute Workout" or this one: "Drinkers Live Longer, According to Science." And don't forget the news that made waves across the country last year: "Drinking Alcohol Makes You a Better Dancer and More Fun at Parties."

In the constant tug-of-war between the you who yearns to be healthy, and the you who yearns to get on

113

the bar and show these peasants what the Macarena should *really* look like, who is right? How can you balance these two and still stay lean for life?

What Alcohol Does to Your Body

Let's clear something up right now. Alcohol is a poison. A delicious, karaoke-enhancing, inhibition decreasing poison.

When you take your first sip for the evening, (or morning, no judgements here), you stimulate GABA receptors in the brain. These, remember, are responsible for relaxing you, which is why alcohol is so good for reducing social anxiety.

The frontal lobe is super susceptible to alcohol, and happens to be the part of the brain that controls social anxiety and decision making. So that's why it's easier to make conversation with that bombshell at the bar who you would never approach at noon.

But while alcohol is swimming around in your brain making you feel good, relaxed, and helping you decide that yes, you do want to sing "It's My Life" by Bon Jovi, it's wreaking havoc on the rest of your body.

Since alcohol is a poison, it causes your body to switch from its normal day-to-day activities of filtering out toxins, metabolizing fats, doing digestion stuff, and giving you erections at inopportune times, to a full-out, code-red emergency mode.

Your body puts all non-essential functions on the back burner and diverts all energy to cleansing you of the toxic waste you just ingested. This is all well and good when you're having a very conservative 1 beer per hour, but when you hit your body with 2 shots of Jägermeister in 60 seconds before following it up with vodka-Red Bulls, shit can really hit the fan.

Instead of metabolizing all the calories you eat and drink normally, your body starts storing those calories as fat while it does everything in its power to keep you alive.

Alcohol technically has 7 calories per gram, but you can't store these calories, because like I said before, it's poison and your body hates it.

But those nachos? That cranberry juice? Those thick, dark beers? All the calories are going STRAIGHT to the place you'd least like to see them. Love handles, belly, thighs? Your body is not without a sick sense of humor.

When you drink:

- You retain more fat from food and drinks than you would have without alcohol.
- You make worse food choices due to lower inhibitions.

- You sleep worse because alcohol makes it harder to get deep REM sleep.
- You have less energy due to the lack of sleep
- You get dehydrated, which decreases energy and can lead to massive loss of strength in the gym
- Full-weekend hangovers are not conducive to an active lifestyle.
- And stop with this "drinking in moderation" thing. Don't derail your progress over two glasses of wine per night.

How to Keep Drinking While Losing Fat

You're not reading this to get chastised for your bad habits, though. You're looking for a practical solution you can integrate into your life to help you do your best in the real world, not some magical fitness-first universe where everyone drinks kombucha and wears leggings to work.

NATE'S HOT TIP

If you drink every night, you WILL NEVER lose fat.

Here's how to get away with drinking while in a fat loss or maintenance phase.

1. Eliminate that glass of wine with dinner
If you're going to drink, do it with friends or loved ones to maximize your lifestyle gains (which are important!), but having small amounts of

alcohol daily is detrimental to your goals of being healthy, lean, and strong.

Rule: Drink twice per week MAX.

2. Say NO to caloric mixers
Don't drink anything with a lot of extra sugar or carbohydrates. Examples of this are Long Island Iced Teas, beer, champagne, and pina coladas.

Instead find a drink that you like that is made from a nice alcohol (no plastic bottles) and doesn't have any calories if you're having a mixed drink. Good examples are Vodka with Soda Water and Lime, Gin and Diet Tonic, or straight alcohol (if you're a scotch drinker).

Rule: Don't drink any calories with your alcohol.

3. Avoid the hangover
Hangovers are caused mostly by dehydration and electrolyte washout from urinating a lot, and to a lesser extent by decreasing your brain chemicals through the magic of drinking too much and having a massive serotonin dump during the night.

To avoid a hangover, follow up each drink with a glass of water, and have another 32 ounces of water before bed, along with a multivitamin, an electrolyte replacement, and Vitamin C.

Rule: Drink a 1:1 alcohol-to-water ratio. Replenish vitamins and minerals before bed.

SUPPLEMENT GUIDE

It's pretty much impossible to get 100 percent of the nutrients you need from the food you eat when you're traveling. Going out to eat will never be able to give you the vitamins and minerals you get from making a green smoothie and some zucchini noodles at home.

To combat that, here are some nutritional supplements that will keep you in good health even while you're on the road.

Do I need to be taking supplements?

Short and douchey answer: "No, you should be eating all perfect food all the time and scrubbing your hands with organic Chernobyl-grade bleach if you so much as brush up against a GMO apple."

That's dumb, and in a country where the supplement industry is raking in a staggering 36 BILLION dollars per year, there's a pretty good chance you have bought, or will buy, supplements in your lifetime.

So what supplements should I take?

HIGH PRIORITY

Protein powder. We talked ad nauseum earlier about the importance of getting enough protein during your day to stay full, fuel your muscles, and promote fat loss. Often, it's hard to get enough on the road, which is why I recommend a protein supplement.

Make sure you get a high-quality "whey protein isolate," which is one of the most bio-available types of protein for the money you're spending. It's a good way to add a quick, satiating meal to your day, especially if you're on the go. It's also a great way to take in more high-quality nutrients when trying to add muscle, and adding protein throughout the day will keep you full and burning fat - even between workouts.

If you find that you get hungry after having a protein shake, you might want to upgrade your game to a meal-replacement shake. This is simply a protein shake with additional ingredients to help satisfy hunger and more accurately replicate the nutrients from a full meal. These also are thicker, which keep you full longer.

Take it:

· *As a meal replacement, or between meal snack.*
· *Post workout*

Vitamin C. You probably don't get enough of this, and it's good for everything from boosting your immune system to helping you recover after a hard workout. Vitamin C can also keep you scurvy free, which is important if your hobbies include raiding, pillaging, and making wenches walk the plank.

119

NATE'S HOT TIP

Put your vitamins near your toothbrush so that you remember in the morning or evening to take them. I'm making the assumption that you do brush your teeth daily.

Take it:

- *In the morning or evening.*

Vitamin D. You don't get enough of this. Doctors in Pacific Northwest don't even test for deficiency anymore, because they were just like, "Yeah, there's a 100 percent chance you're deficient. Buy Vitamin D pills, take 5000 ius per day. Next!"

If you're feeling sick, you can take 10,000-15,000 drops or 2-3 pills, to help keep the immune system strong enough to fight off a bug.

Take it:

- *In the morning with breakfast.*

Fish oil. While our modern diet is riddled with Omega-6's which can cause more inflammation, we don't get enough Omega-3's, which prevent inflammation and keep our bodies functioning at a high level. It's important to try to get a 2:1 ratio of Omega-3 to Omega-6, but the typical North American diet promotes the exact opposite.

Getting a high-quality fish oil supplement can help fix that, in addition to all of the other benefits: bone strength, hair sheen, general healing, skin quality, eye health, heart health, more insulin sensitivity, and clearer mental focus.

Take it:

- *Twice per day, with breakfast and dinner.*

MEDIUM PRIORITY

Branched-Chain Amino Acids (BCAAs). BCAAs can help you hold on to muscle mass while eating at a caloric deficit or while fasting. Protein will break down into amino acids in the stomach and small intestine, but has a higher calorie count, which makes BCAAs ideal for fasting, or any time you want to train without spiking your blood sugar.

They aren't necessary, but since they're sweet and you can drink them 2-3 times per day, BCAAs also help cut down on cravings.

Take it:

- *Between meals, 2-3 times per day. Before training while fasting.*

Zinc/Magnesium/Melatonin. These both boost growth hormone and testosterone levels to help with recovery. They also help with getting deeper, more restful sleep.

These can give you weird dreams, but are very helpful for increasing feelings of sleepiness before bed time.

And even if the supplements themselves don't do a lot for hormonal balance, the better you sleep, the more balanced your hormones will be.

Take it:

- *Before bed. Don't exceed recommended dose.*

Probiotics. Gut health is one of the most overlooked pieces of overall heath-and-recovery abilities. You can get probiotics by eating fermented foods like kimchee, sauerkraut, or kefir – or by eating papaya seeds, which I believe cured many a jungle-related disease I may have been susceptible to.

If you take antibiotics, it's always a good practice to take a probiotic to help bring back some of the good bacteria to help you break down and digest food, in addition to playing a major role in building back up the immune system.

Find these in the refrigerated section, or just use the foods above, especially when you're on the road.

Take it:

- *With a meal, twice per day*

Pre workouts. I love a good pre-workout supplement, but keep in mind that you're not getting "new" energy, you're simply borrowing it from later. That's why it's not great to take energy supplements (including coffee) daily. Give your body a bit of time to recover a couple days per week.

The major effective ingredient in every pre workout is caffeine, so when companies say they have a "proprietary blend" it's usually a mix of taurine, guarine, beta alanine (the tingly sensation you get if you take too much also prevents fatigue in muscles), and some form of creatine (to enhance the pump).

Just FYI, when a label says "proprietary blend" what it means is, "We don't have to tell you anything we put in here, so it might be 95 percent cat dander and 5 percent crystal meth. Go on, try it. You'll like it."

Take it:

- *15 minutes before your workout.*

Greens supplement. Most of us have a hard time getting all our servings of fruits and veggies when we're at home, so it can be especially important to bring a green supplement with you when traveling for a while.

It's like insurance. A green juice a good way to get the phytonutrients to stay healthy and prevent inflammation from training, poor eating habits, and day-to-day activities.

Take it:

- *In your breakfast shake.*

- *Before bed – I like to mix in a packet of Emergen-C for flavor and a Vitamin C boost.*

LOW PRIORITY (AKA: DON'T TAKE THIS GARBAGE)

Weight-gainer powder/shakes. This is the biggest scam in the supplement world. Low-quality protein is combined with low-quality carbohydrates (mostly coming from some compound that is basically pure sugar) and companies slap a label on it that shows some monster bench-pressing 900 pounds before eating a full bison.

Take this instead:

- *3 extra peanut butter and jelly sandwiches on top of your normal diet.*

Fat burners – On the opposite side of the scam coin, you'll know these by the lithe sensual female wearing booty shorts and looking over her shoulder in a surprised, "Who, me?" expression.

Most of these products have ingredients similar to pre workouts, which means that caffeine plays a strong role. Some other offenders: green coffee-bean extract, raspberry ketones, and Garcinia Cambogia.

They can help a bit as caffeine causes a slight uptick in overall body heat and heart rate, both which burn small amounts of extra calories. Additionally, caffeine is an appetite suppressant, and can arguably help you control cravings.

Take This Instead:

- *Coffee in the morning, and if you need a boost in the afternoon, switch to green tea.*

Garcinia Cambogia/raspberry ketones. Can we just move forward and agree that as a country we will stop buying supplements that we see on TV?

Unfortunately the answer is "Yeah! We'll definitely sto— Wait, did you say I could lose 10 pounds in 3 days?!?!?"

Take This Instead:

- *Cigarettes. It's hard to eat when you're smoking.*

Section 9: Training

I know it's late in the book to finally start answering the question, "Why did you put fitness in the title of the book if we're never going to talk about training?"

Ok, fine, here it is, but I just had a lot of stuff I wanted to get off my chest about hydration. Hope you enjoyed it. If you skipped all the rest of the book and are finally joining us here, welcome! It's great to have you.

In the "Why You Should Care" section there was much talk about how consistency is the secret ingredient that separates those with the "diet starts tomorrow" mentality from those among us who seem to be perpetually walking around shirtless.

There's a big difference between a great program that was put together by a coach with experience and a deep knowledge of the human body, and a program that your friend Brian found in a 1997 version of "Muscle and Fitness" that recommends 90 minutes of biceps three times per week.

But the principle of consistency tells us that even a crummy program done habitually will yield better results than an amazing program done, "whenever you're feeling up to it."

A great program will also complement whatever else is going on in your life. If you're a new dad with a job that involves you taking 30-plus business trips per year, training six times per week for 90 minutes at a time probably isn't reasonable, and trying to "gut it out" and stick to an impossible program is going to end in frustration rather than results.

If travel is a major part of your lifestyle, it's necessary to find a style of training that works in a park or hotel room that can be done in a short amount of time with maximum efficiency.

You might have a personal trainer at home, and love sweating your balls off in hot yoga. Or maybe there's a spin instructor whose class (and tight spandex) keeps you coming back. It can be hard to replicate your favorite style of training at home, so it's important to have the ability to get in a good workout wherever you are, and on your terms.

Essential equipment

When I travel, I like to take a few pieces of training equipment with me that fit in a carry on and have multiple uses. The more versatile the better, but I'll change what I bring depending on where I'm going and what my program entails at the time.

BEST TRAVEL-TRAINING EQUIPMENT

Suspension strap. This one piece is the best thing you can bring with you anywhere. It's small, fits in a backpack or carry on, and can be used to harness your bodyweight to do any exercise and work every muscle group in a unique way.

I have used my suspension strap on top of mountains, in dirty hostel laundry rooms, in a butcher's kitchen, on a children's swing set in the heart of the Andes, on the mast of a boat in the middle of the jungle, and wrapped around a cactus (not my best move).

Suspension straps come with an extender that can be wrapped around vertical or horizontal poles, as well as a door anchor that can be used to transform any regular door into a veritable fitness playground.

The straps are amazing because you can use your body weight as resistance and make it as hard or as easy as you need to challenge yourself. I've trained an 84-year-old client on them, as well as elite-level swimmers, professional golfers, and everyday dudes who just want to look good without bothering that cranky shoulder.

You can easily make the workout harder or easier by adjusting where you're standing in relation to the anchor point of the suspension strap, which is great because as the set progresses and you get more tired, it's simple to just take a step back, and reduce the difficulty of the move. That becomes much harder when you have to set down the weights and go pick up another size.

Suspension straps are just another way to make exercise faster and more efficient, key components of this style of training.

Resistance bands. Bands are great because they can be attached to anything and be used for any exercise that you can do on a $10,000 cable machine. Deadlifts, squats, rows, presses and any combination is possible with the right band and right set up.

When possible, I like to bring the resistance bands and the suspension strap because they're small, and the bands can be used in the door anchor of the suspension strap for a ton of great exercises.

The best bands in the world are latex-based, 40-inch resistance bands – the ones that are a full circle and no plastic handles. These last much longer and can be used for any exercise, while the bands with handles are limited when it comes to many core movements.

If you have to pick one, opt for the half-inch band because it's great for posture and arm exercises. The

1-inch band can provide resistance of up to 120 pounds, so it's better if you're stronger or are looking to increase the difficulty of a squat or a deadlift. Any band bigger than 1 inch isn't necessary for your travel equipment.

Core sliders. Core sliders are basically furniture movers with padding. The best sliders have one side that works on carpet, and then a softer side that works on tile or wood.

These are great for training all aspects of core and lower body, and the exercises are limited only by imagination. The one downfall of the sliders – and the reason why I sometimes won't bring them – is because they aren't useable outside, or on rubber flooring, so if you're staying or training in place with either of those, you might not get as much out of those as you will the other two.

However, they are flat, and easy to pack in a carry on, so it's not hard to bring them with you.

Mini bands. Mini bands are small bands that are 10-12 inches in diameter and can be used for a variety of exercises when wrapped around the feet or hands. They're incredibly small, and can be packed into backpacks or fanny packs, or you could literally just keep them in your back pocket.

But don't let their size deceive you: Mini bands can provide some great exercises for the legs, hips, core

131

and, smaller muscles of the body. Using mini bands to activate the muscles of the hips before a doing a strength move has helped my clients stay pain free, and doing any of these exercises with careful control and precision is guaranteed to make you sweat.

THE TRAINING PROGRAM

All of the above are great tools and can be used to create the lean, healthy body of your dreams, but only if you use them. A hammer, wrench, and drill are also great and can be used to build a house, but only if you know what you're doing, or have a manual to go by.

That's why it's important to have a training program that is innovative, and one that fits your goals and equipment.

In April of 2017, I launched a company that was aimed at doing just that: Providing busy people with the equipment and knowledge to get or stay in the best shape of their life, no matter how demanding their schedule.

Called Bod in a Box, it's the ideal solution for at home or travel training. It comes with a suspension strap, two resistance bands, core sliders, and mini bands, and a daily program that can be done anywhere, with videos explaining the unique bodyweight exercises.

While it's possible to get in great shape without the equipment or program from Bod in a Box (and I'll show you how to create your own training program), I wanted to make the process as easy as possible for people who don't have time to research, build, purchase, and pack their own home gym. If you want to make a lifestyle change, you must be consistent, and the best way to become increasingly consistent is to have everything as easy as possible.

With Bod in a Box, I removed the most common excuses I hear as to why people can't get a good workout on their own – No time, no equipment, and no program.

To learn more, visit bodinabox.com

BODY-WEIGHT TRAINING IS THE ELIXIR OF LIFE.

It might surprise you to find out that some of the most prolific athletes in pro basketball, football and golf are switching their routines from traditional weight lifting to being primarily bodyweight based.

Hundreds of athletes, from NFL quarterback Drew Brees, to Olympic swimmer Christine Magnusson, and UFC athlete Brandon Vera use body-weight exercise as the main portion of their exercise routine.

What's causing this shift from the gym to the park? Is there any merit in taking your training from the weight room to your living room?

Science says YES. Here's why.

BODY-WEIGHT TRAINING BUILDS MORE MUSCLE

The majority of body-weight training is classified as "closed chain." This is the fancy scientific way of saying that you're moving your body through space instead of moving an outside object.

For example, a pullup is closed chain, while a lat pulldown is open chain.

Pushup – closed chain. Bench press – open chain.

Squat – closed chain. Leg press – open chain.

You get the idea.

Who cares?

According to a study by the Journal of Orthopedic and Sports Physical Therapy, closed-chain exercises were responsible for a 31 percent increase in lower body strength after only six weeks, while the open chain group only improved 13 percent.

The body-weight group also saw a marked increase in power output, increasing vertical-jump capabilities by 10 percent while there was no increase in the machine-based group.

By learning to move your own body though space, you increase the amount of muscle fibers used. This directly causes more strength and muscular gains.

And if you're at the level where you can do push-ups and pullups all day without it being challenging, just add some extra "bodyweight" in the form of a weight vest or chains.

BODY-WEIGHT TRAINING BURNS MORE FAT

Imagine this. You and your caveman buddies are out foraging for berries, looking at rocks, and cracking jokes, when all the sudden a sabre-tooth tiger snatches up your friend Grog!

The rest of your group scatters, climbing trees to escape the tiger.

During this scenario your body is in fight-or-flight mode, dumping adrenaline into your bloodstream to help you escape. It's also demanding that you release your non-functional tissue (fat), and instead prioritizing functional tissue (muscle). This is to ensure that you're able to climb a tree faster and save your life.

Doing body-weight exercises triggers an evolutionary mechanism in your body and brain that makes your body release fat. Our bodies only understand stress, they don't know that you're doing pullups at a comfortable gym with some Justin Bieber on the speakers, they only know you're pulling yourself up, away from danger. Probably trying to escape a T-Rex or something. Classic.

WHY IS THIS IMPORTANT?

Even though your workouts aren't technically life or death, your body only knows stress – so when you activate your sympathetic nervous system and initiate that fight or flight response through training, using bodyweight training signals your body to release fat to keep you alive.

That's why a pullup will always be a better option than a pulldown. You use more muscle, burn more calories, and improve your hormonal signaling to burn fat.

If your goal is fat loss, the more you can move your body, the better results you'll get. Get off that machine and start using a suspension strap.

Even if the bench press is reserved for you every Monday from 4-6 p.m., and you'd rather get diabetes than give up your beloved leg press, your muscle mass and fat loss would both benefit from adding some additional closed-chain exercise.

HOW DO I ADD IN MORE BODY-WEIGHT TRAINING?

Adding more bodyweight training is easy.

If you already use the gym on a regular basis, just substitute some of your current machine or weighted exercises for body-weight versions of the same muscle group.

Pushing. Push-ups/pike push-ups/single-arm push-ups

Pulling. Suspension-trainer row/chin-ups/one-arm row

Legs. Squats/lunges/rear-leg elevated split squats/jump squat

Adding in just a few minutes of home-based exercise per day has been shown to be an effective way to achieve long-term results, as well as build the habits needed to stay lean for life.

Bod in a Box comes with a great program based around body-weight exercise and can be used if you literally only have 15 minutes per day to workout, or if you have a bit more time. It also has some of the most effective training programs in the world, which is why Bod in a Box is the best 30-minute workout in the world.

Use Bod in a Box's programming principles to create your own amazing workout.

YOUR FORMULA FOR CREATING AN AMAZING WORKOUT

1. Short circuit

Any time we're training with time constraints OR trying to lose fat, it's very important to work out in a circuit fashion. This simply means repeating 2-4 exercises in a row. This helps us stay efficient and effective, which are very important especially if you are limited to a short workout.

Technically, a "superset" is two consecutive exercises. A "circuit" is two or more exercises done in order, then repeated for the given amount of sets.

Training this way can also give your muscles a bit of a break while continuing to tax your lungs and heart. If you're working your upper body, rather than doing a set of push-ups and then waiting 60 seconds before repeating them, it's much more efficient to do a set of rows between.

It's a totally different muscle group, so the chest and triceps still get the 60-second break from the push-ups, but your body never stops moving. This is important for burning fat.

Rule: Always cycle through 2-4 different exercises, and keep moving.

2. Warm it up

The first circuit or superset shouldn't be the hardest. Instead, it should be carefully chosen movements that prepare your joints, tendons, and ligaments for the rigor of the workout.

If you're going to do an upper-body workout, the first circuit should help warm up your shoulders and upper body until they're feeling good and slightly "pumped." A great warmup always helps to fill the muscles with blood, which keeps them warm and protects the joints. A great upper-body warm up could be:

Suspension strap rows x 60 seconds (shoulders, back, and biceps)

Suspension strap fallouts x 60 seconds (front of shoulders, triceps, and core)

Avoid rest during the warmup sets. If you are gassed after your warmups, they're either too hard, or you need to work out more.

Rule: The first circuit should warm you up and prepare you for the workout.

3. Eat your meat

Everyone knows you can't have any pudding if you don't eat your meat. Likewise, you shouldn't just jump into an ab finisher without first doing the "meat" of your workout.

139

The second circuit should be the most important piece of the workout, especially if you're pressed for time.

These exercises should be compound, which means they should involve more than one joint and muscle group. This means you want to save your bicep curls for later and first do a pullup, because that hits the back, shoulders and biceps. The second circuit can be between 2-4 exercises.

Rule: Do the biggest exercises in the second circuit, and save the isolation exercises for later.

4. Count to 10

When choosing exercises for your circuits, especially the "meat" of your workout, it's tempting to add in all the hard exercises you can think of. But doing a workout that looks like this:

Suspension-strap Bulgarian split squat

Suspension-strap burpee

Pull-up

... is a good way to get wrecked after just one round. We want to be able to recover enough to get through the circuit for the prescribed number of rounds, so sometimes we need to tone down the intensity. That's why I use the Rule of 10. I like to think of an exercise on a scale from 1 (easy mode) to 10 (brb gotta kneel next to the toilet for a minute).

If you start off with an exercise that's a 7/10 like Bulgarian split squats, you want to follow it up with an exercise that's a 3, like band pull-aparts, or a plank.

Make sure to challenge yourself without taking it all the way to the danger zone – it's not great when you have to postpone a client meeting because you can't get your heart rate back down below 130.

Rule: Make sure your exercises add up to a '10' difficulty by combining harder exercises with easier ones.

5. Rest > everything
When training for fat loss, or doing a body-weight training program, the most important variable you can manipulate is your rest time. If the allotted rest time is only 30 seconds but you're finding that you need 90 to recover from the exercise, cut back the intensity of the exercise so that you're recovered within the 30 seconds.

This means moving your body away from the anchor point so it's less difficult, or adding an easier move in the middle to get a short "active" rest. Either way, adhering to rest times is the most effective way to get a great workout in a short amount of time.

Try not to rest at all in the middle of a circuit when moving between exercises.

For maximum fat loss, rest for 45 seconds or less after each circuit. For muscle building, rest 75 seconds or less after each circuit, and for maximum strength (think: 1 rep max deadlift), rest 3-5 minutes.

Rule: Don't rest between exercises; rest less than 45 seconds between circuits for max fat loss.

6. Finish him!

If you're not crunched for time, a finisher is a great way to get the most out of your workout and make sure that you're continually progressing. Finishers are circuits done at the end of a workout that are difficult, allow you to work to your limit, and can be used for really finishing off the body part you used during the workout, or for adding in a little bit more volume of a weak movement.

Many people like to do abdominal exercises as a finisher because they feel that their core needs more training. Either way, this is when you should really be pushing yourself as hard as possible and working to your limit.

Many people find it easier to make that big push since they know that they're only a few minutes from being completely done.

Rule: Create a circuit that can be done intensely and works on a weak area or body part to maximize your finisher.

EXAMPLE WORKOUT

Here's an example workout that I do with Bod in a Box users that takes advantage of all the principles listed above. It would be easy to write another book strictly on training principles and how to write an effective program, but I've found the best way is by doing effective programs written by knowledgeable coaches and tweaking little things to adapt it to my specific needs.

Experience is the best teacher, so keep practicing by showing up and being consistent with your workouts. If you don't want to spend the time researching and writing your own program, visit BodinaBox.com to sign up for a proven training program that will get you results in less than 30 minutes per day.

Shoulder Skorcher

Complete ALL exercises in a circuit and then rest for indicated length before repeating circuit or moving to next circuit.

Notes:		

EXPRESS WORKOUT		
Band Pull Apart		60 Sec
Bodyweight Plank Shoulder Taps		60 Sec
	Number Of Rounds:	2
	Rest After Each Round:	0 Sec

Notes:		

EXPRESS WORKOUT		
Suspension Trainer Row		40 Sec
Suspension Trainer Pushup		40 Sec
	Number Of Rounds:	3
	Rest After Each Round:	30 Sec

Notes:		

EXTENDED WORKOUT		
Suspension Trainer Rear Delt Flies		30 Sec
Band Single Arm Row		30 Sec Ea
Suspension Trainer Triceps Extension		30 Sec
	Number Of Rounds:	4
	Rest After Each Round:	30 Sec

Notes:		

FINSHER		
Jog		1/2 Mile
	Number Of Rounds:	
	Rest After Each Round:	

The first two circuits will take about 15 minutes if there's no down time between exercises or rounds. Those are the circuits in the "express" workout. Designed to warm up and hit the meat and potatoes of the workout before getting on with your life. If this is all you do, it's still a successful workout.

The third circuit is the extended workout. This will take you to about 24 minutes. This is where we do a little bit more volume on the lower body, which was the focus for the day.

The finisher is a light jog that will take a couple minutes if you have the time, and will leave you feeling strong and healthy – perfect for the start to a busy day on the road or in meetings.

This whole workout should be done in 40 minutes or less (27 if followed exactly) and will give you better results than 99 percent of other workouts on the planet. It's a perfect blend of strength, cardio, and core training to have you looking and feeling your best.

The exercises might be named something confusing that you don't understand, which is why they're all linked to video explanations when you get the program delivered to your email, so even though it might be hard to figure out what a "band single arm row" is in this medium, it's much easier with a Bod in a Box clickable video library at your fingertips.

You can use the tips above to create your own version of this, but there are thousands of books written on writing great programs, so there's always more to learn.

Ok, I'm finished shamelessly plugging my product. I just think it's awesome, and will make your life easier.

Onward!

THE MOTIVATION TRAP

Too many people have told me they weren't able to get their workouts in because they lack the motivation to do it.

To hear many people talk about it, motivation sounds a lot like cash. You grab the stuff you want, go to check out, reach into your pocket and, oh no! You're fresh out of motivation. Now you gotta pretend like you left your wallet in your car and just leave the store.

But walk into their workplace and you'll find them working hard at finding and submitting reports that they're probably not motivated to do either.

What's the difference?

Motivation infers that there is an option.

If you asked 100 people with jobs, all 100 would say that they *HAVE TO* go to work. It's not dependent on whether they're feeling like it. You work, or you don't eat. It's simple.

When you can reach this same level with your morning routine and your training habits, that's when the results start taking care of themselves.

When fitness becomes a "must do" rather than a "should do," you rid yourself of the need for motivation.

146

Here are four ways to get past motivation and become and stay fit – for life.

PRINCIPLE 1: THE 5-MINUTE RULE

If you ever have a big task that needs to be done, but it sounds like the last thing that you would like to do, force yourself to start the task and do **ONLY** 5 minutes' worth of work. Whether that's sitting down to write a few sentences of an article you've been putting off, cleaning a room, or doing your homework, often it takes just 5 minutes to get into a rhythm and find your flow.

Sometimes after 5 minutes, you're so engrossed in the task that you find it easy to finish. But even if you're still feeling bogged down after those 5 minutes, get up, walk away, and try another 5 minutes later on.

Application: Put on the clothes

If you need to get up earlier to train or run, and those sound like the furthest thing from what you want to do on a cold morning, tell yourself that all you need to do is get out of bed and put on your workout clothes and shoes.

It's much easier if these are already out, visible, and you don't need to go rooting around in your closet to find them. Once you're up and dressed, the temptation to go back to bed is much less.

147

Principle 2: Temptation coupling

Temptation coupling is simply pairing one stimulus that you've been putting off – like working out, cleaning the house, or working on a big project – with a positive stimulus, like listening to an addictive audio book, eating a donut, or buying a new toy.

A study by Katherine Milkman, a professor at The Wharton School, showed that participants were 40 percent more likely to go the gym if they had an interesting audio book to listen to while they were there. Those efforts increased to 60 percent if they were prohibited from listening to the audio book outside of the gym.

Application: Enjoy the gym with a good book or music

When you hit the gym, have a reward system in place. (**Hint:** a donut isn't the best option). If you have a great new album that you want to listen to, or you're in the middle of a highly addictive book that you don't allow yourself to finish outside of the gym, that positive stimulus will be enough to push you past any initial hesitations.

If you hit the gym 10 times in 2 weeks, buy those new shoes or workout pants you want, and then only wear them when you're exercising. Anything to pair fun activity with something that you're not as thrilled to do.

Principle 3: Accountability

In my personal experience, clients who are made accountable to finish their program are four times more likely to follow through with exercise, which makes this an extremely powerful principle.

Having a coach to report back to makes it harder to justify that third gin and tonic when you haven't finished all your workouts for the week.

Application: Have a plan

If you know that each week, there are 5 workouts that you must complete in 7 days, that reduces the need for willpower to get you to the gym, because now it's not a question of "if" you'll get the workouts done, but rather "when." This change in mentality is small, but makes a huge difference in your perception and behavior.

Even though buying a program can seem like an unnecessary cost (especially when your gym offers classes), the benefit in terms of motivation is easily worth the cost. And that doesn't even include the muscular development that you'll get from following a carefully laid-out training program.

Principle 4: Scheduling

When you have a 9:30 a.m. meeting with a client, you know what you need to do to make it there. Showered and fed by 8:30, out the door by 9, puts you at their office by 9:25 with a 5-minute buffer to look for a parking space or deal with traffic.

Those of us who have jobs and wish to keep them don't think about motivation as being a factor in getting our work done. That should be the same attitude you take toward your body, which loves you very much and wants the best for you.

Application: Set a time

Go to your calendar and schedule out your workouts for the week. Have a clear start and end time, and use that time to do your training session. If you only have time to workout between 7-7:30 a.m., you'll be more likely to use that time effectively because it's finite and already scheduled in your day.

Remember ...

Not every principle is a great fit for everyone. Try out several of them and see which works better for your brain and your schedule.

Don't forget that health and fitness isn't a 6-week journey to a bikini body – it's a lifelong endeavor, and thus doesn't have to be perfect tomorrow. If we are improving every day, we will eventually win.

Section 10: Wrap-Up

I hope you had fun reading this book. To a lesser extent, I hope you learned some good stuff that you can start applying to your every-day life, especially if you find yourself trapped in an airline seat more than once per month.

Remember the Bruce Lee quote from the beginning of the book? "Take what is useful, discard what is not." That's the mental process I hope you went through when reading: Mining for little nuggets of good information and quickly discarding all the rude stuff I said about accounting, cats, and wearing pants.

Remember...

Exercise is a necessary part of life if you want to look great, feel good, and have energy for the things you love, like hanging out with your kids, and long PowerPoint presentations. If you don't feel great, the rest of your life just becomes harder.

The sooner you get into a consistent habit of exercising, the sooner you'll get good at this new skill, and the sooner you'll enjoy it. And if you don't enjoy it, hey, too damn bad.

I don't enjoy flossing, but I enjoy smiling and not getting cavities filled, so I do it anyway.

The most effective type of training if you're low on time or looking to burn body fat is bodyweight training. Cardio burns calories, lifting heavy builds strength, but bodyweight training triggers an evolutionary mechanism in your brain that will increase lean muscle and decrease body fat. Have you ever seen an obese person do 15 pull-ups?

Body-weight training will also help you feel better, move better, and have more energy for the day. It truly is the elixir of life, and learning how to harness it effectively is one more step in getting a Ph.D. in your own body.

Add body-weight training to your gym workouts, or simply start a program based on these scientific principles for maximum results. Even 10 minutes per day as part of a morning routine can be powerful for body and brain, and will provide you with a huge return on the time investment.

Please Stop...

... Googling "best diet for fat loss," "Kardashian superfoods," or "how much weight will I lose if I only eat lemons."

This book contains plenty of nutritional nuggets to help you hit your goals as well as actionable tips to keep you from binging on the road or setting your progress back while on vacation.

There are tons of fancy diets and supplements out there that promise great results in days, but those kinds of results don't last. I got some great advice from a homeless man in Ecuador who told me that, "If it sounds too good to be true, it probably is." He went on to tell me that the government was harboring aliens that looked like centaurs and that you only need to eat aloe vera to survive, so take that with a grain of salt.

The big rocks of nutrition are:

Hydration. Always.

Eat protein with every meal. No protein? No meal.

Avoid alcohol, especially while you eat.

Eat ingredients as much as possible.

If you can do these four things 90 percent of the time, you're on the right path to change your body, keep your energy high, and stay healthy for as long as you're on this earth.

In conclusion...

Remember your why. You don't travel because you just love the conference room in the Boston Marriott. We travel for our jobs, our family, our lifestyle. For fun, for sun, for adventure. And yes, because if we didn't travel we would probably get fired.

While I was working as a tour guide in the Panamanian jungle for a crazy ex-marine named Carl he often threatened to fire me and feed my body to jungle animals if I didn't adhere to the rules of the vessel. These rules included:

Get up early to paddleboard and look for birds.

Drink with Captain Carl on the top deck at night and look at the stars.

Wear a shirt at dinner.

Oh yea, and catch crocodiles for tourists out of the river on the night safari.

It was something that Carl would throw in my face regularly during the first few months aboard. He like to tell me about an Australian guy (obviously he was an aussie) that would literally jump out of the boat at night to wrestle crocodiles in the river.

Eventually some friends came to visit to see if we truly were alive in Panama or if we had been killed months ago and our bodies used to move massive quantities of cocaine. I had finally had enough of Captain Carl's shit, (and enough rum) that when we went out on the river at night, I felt like I had lived a long and productive enough life that if I were to die, it would probably be fine.

The boat started up with me at the front, a massive 1000-watt floodlight in hand. We slowly cruised up the river looking for nocturnal animals. If you stand directly behind the flashlight, when the light hits an animal's eyes, they shine back at you. Blue for mammals, white or green for birds, and red for reptiles.

As we turned a bend in the river, I noticed a large set of red eyes on the opposite side of the river. We killed the motor and drifted slowly up towards a big Spectacled Caiman. A Spectacled Caiman is basically a crocodile with a shorter snout and big rings around it's eyes that make it look like it's wearing glasses.

Just the eyes and tip of his nose were above water, but I could tell he was larger than average. I remember thinking "ok, I've been training daily for weeks, and all this son of a bitch has been doing is swimming around biting shit". Then, without truly pondering the long-term consequences of my actions – I jumped.

I landed in the murky water with my hands around his neck, and both my legs around his tail and lower *body. After a brief struggle that included a frantic roll over escape attempt and violent tail thrashing, I was able to hold on to what eventually was revealed to be a 5-foot long water dinosaur. In my jubilee and with several gallons of adrenaline coursing through my rum infused blood stream, I crawled back onto the boat, holding the neck of the caiman for dear life.*

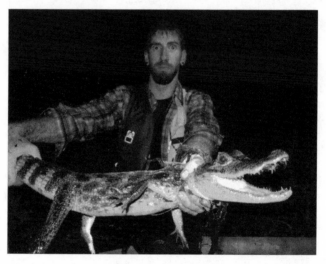

While I don't recommend catching a caiman simply to prove that you're in shape, it's important to remember that nothing is worth doing if you're miserable.

Inject your life with the benefits that being fit and healthy can bring, and reap the rewards of a healthy body, strong mind, and energy to pursue your passions, even when they include insane activities like crocodile wrestling, and preparing for the zombie apocalypse.

If not, well hey, there's always the Cotton Ball Diet.

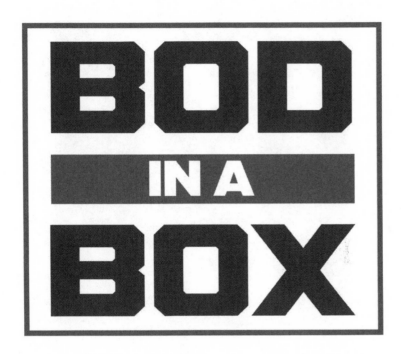

To get a FREE copy of the workout program that I've used successfully with hundreds of clients, visit:

http://bodinabox.com/free

Learn:

- The home workout you can do anywhere
- The best exercises you can do in a hotel room
- The right pace for a 15-minute workout that will give you results
- The one exercise you need to be doing every day